WHY YOUR BODY PREFERS PLANTS

The Science-Backed Path to Health, Energy, and Longevity

The Plant Diet Book

by

Robert Enochs

About the Author

Thank You for considering my book. The storm of information you're about to read is going to sound incredible at times, but I would like to invite you to stay the course and brave these rough waters with me.

Robert Enochs has followed a plant-based lifestyle for decades, spending years studying nutrition, human biology, and the long-term health effects of modern diets. After witnessing firsthand how deeply diet influences energy, inflammation, and overall well-being, he wrote this book to explore *why* the human body responds so strongly to plant-based foods.

Rather than promoting trends or ideology, Robert focuses on evidence, anatomy, and critical thinking—encouraging readers to question common assumptions about food and health. His goal is simple: to help people better understand what they eat, why it matters, and how informed choices can lead to lasting wellness.

Contents

Introduction: Plant Power - Unveiling a Healthier You

Imagine the very core of your well-being, the energy that fuels your day, and the vitality that colors your life could all be radically transformed by the choices you make at the dining table.

We've been on a collective journey, some of us tracing the steps of our ancestors, while others have been caught up in the lies and propaganda of the latest trends and mainstream narratives. Many of us have attempted to uncover the diet secret that best suits our modern lives whilst staying true to our evolutionary makeup. Many more have been totally clueless about what we are eating and what it is actually doing to our bodies.

What we're uncovering, time and time again, is the powerful truth that a Plant-Based Diet holds the key to unlocking a healthier you. Sure, we all know that we need to "eat healthy and exercise" - but what does "eat healthy" actually mean? We have all been lied to about what eating healthy means, starting with the consumption of animal proteins, fast foods, and others, to the point where most Americans have no idea how to eat right.

Some of these lies are born out of necessity, like fast food or highly processed foods, for example, and other lies are based on ignorance (albeit not always intentional in every instance).

Habits and cultural norms often dictate a plate centered around meat, but what if I told you that leafy greens, vibrant vegetables, and hearty grains could not only match but potentially surpass the touted benefits of meat consumption?

The narrative of protein-packed meat being the pinnacle of nutrition is being rewritten by the potent potential of plant-based diets. The evidence is mounting, not just in clinical studies but in the personal triumphs of those who've turned over a new leaf, showing us that plants can offer a symphony of nutrients that work in concert to elevate our health.

This introduction serves as the gateway to understanding how embracing a diet rich in plants is not just about abstaining from meat but about proactively choosing a lifestyle that is aligned with your body's natural tendencies.

Let's embark on a transformative journey together, one seedling at a time, as we uncover the overwhelming evidence and the ageless wisdom that will nudge you toward an existence brimming with health. It's not mere hyperbole to say that a plant-based diet can change your life - it's a growing reality for people around the globe, and it starts with the simple yet profound decision to let plants power your path to wellness.

Chapter 1: A Brief History of Human Diet

The story of the human diet is, in many ways, a tale of adaptation and survival.

The argument about when humans first arrived is debatable, but most of us can agree that the earliest human civilizations first began around equatorial regions where the planet is warm.

It is my understanding that our early ancestors began life here on the planet around the "Fertile Crescent" along the Tigris and Euphrates rivers in Mesopotamia (now modern-day Iraq). We don't know exactly when early hominids got there, and we don't know when they began to migrate away from that area.

But, in 2001, archaeologists discovered 'Sahelanthropus tchadensis' (known as Toumaï). They found nine specimens in the Djurab Desert of northern Chad, Africa, and believe them to be roughly **7 million years old**. Toumaï represents one of the earliest known members of the hominid family and provides valuable insights into the early stages of human history and what they ate.

Yes, I know – the Earth isn't that old, but stay with me here.

The year prior, in 2000, archaeologists discovered 'Orrorin Tugenensis', which is believed to be roughly 6 million years old. This discovery was made in Kenya,

Africa, and as of 2007, 20 specimens of Orrorin Tugenensis have been found.

Some archeologists speculate that the earliest known ancestors of hominoids (the species of apes and humans) began as early as 23-34 million years ago, but let's stick with actual hominid remains that have been discovered.

These early human-like animals discovered in 2000-2001 lived sometime between six and seven million years ago in West-Central Africa, walked upright, and had ape-like or human-like features. Some features include small canine teeth "and a spinal cord opening underneath the skull instead of towards the back as seen in non-bipedal apes." If you want to read more about this animal, please visit https://humanorigins.si.edu/evidence/human-fossils/species/sahelanthropus-tchadensis

The Smithsonian website continues: Because the teeth were heavily worn from age, they have yet to fully understand the isotopes that would indicate diet, but they "...can infer based on its environment and other early human species that it ate a mainly plant-based diet."

It's impossible to know what these early hominids had for lunch with only a handful of bone fragments, but we have a couple of sources we can look at for an idea of what they might have eaten. First, we have the Christian Bible as a possible source to suggest what the first man (and woman) ate in the Garden of Eden. This would have been a strict plant-based diet if you believe the Bible.

If you're not a Bible believer, then we can only speculate what they ate. A second source we can look at (for what early humans ate) is the tens of thousands of Sumerian clay tablets discovered in Uruk (southern Mesopotamia). But the problem here is that these Cuneiform tablets are only about 5,200 years old, and they only tell us what the Sumerians were eating at that time – not what early hominids ate millions of years ago.

Regardless, the Cuneiform tablets tell us what they ate. The Sumerians were civilized and heavy into agriculture, so it was essentially a plant-based diet, but they did eat meat, too.

People of Sumer enjoyed beans, onions, lentils, chickpeas, garlic, leeks, cucumber, cress, mustard spice, green lettuce, and they used goat's milk. They ate eggs for breakfast, raised pigs, and fished. Tablets also indicate they traded wild fowl, deer, goat, chicken, and venison.

The most important aspect of all this was that meat was only supplemental - it was not the primary food source. Animals were expensive and in short supply, so they used them wisely – it was nowhere near the meat consumption of today's American culture.

'In The Beginning' (according to the Bible) was a plant-based diet, but as hominids moved away from the Tigris and Euphrates rivers in Mesopotamia (and more toward the grasslands of Africa and the colder climates of Europe and Asia), necessity dictated more meat in their diets, and animal hides to keep them warm.

Now, as I just stated a moment ago, the first hominid was believed to have been here 6 – 7 million years ago, so we can only speculate what this early human-like animal ate. We will talk more about the physiology of a primate in the coming chapters to make it crystal clear what these early humans probably ate, but for now, let's assume they ate whatever they could find.

I'm sure they foraged for nuts, berries, and fruit and sometimes even scavenged a freshly killed animal carcass occasionally, as nature provided. Keep in mind that they did not yet have tools or weapons to hunt with until millions of years later (if you believe in science).

Understand that running down an animal to hunt and kill by bludgeoning it to death with stones is tremendously hard work (if not impossible) for most hominids and primates.

Hominids, like modern humans (without tools), do not have claws or sharp teeth to rip their prey apart or tear its hide and flesh loose from the body and bones.

Just imagine trying to run down a rabbit or deer, and then if by some miracle you were able to catch and beat it to death with a stone – imagine trying to bite into the hide with your teeth to rip the flesh and fur into manageable chunks? It is impossible for hominids or humans to do this on a regular basis without tools, and they would have gone extinct.

Speaking of tools, it is a fact that early humans did use tools to kill and process animals, but that came millions of years later, as far as we know. Stay with me here and think this through.

Take a look at this chart for a better understanding of the timeline.

- 7 million years ago - Sahelanthropus tchadensis, known as Toumaï emerges in Africa

- 6 million years ago - Orrorin Tugenensis emerges in East Africa.

- 4.4 million years ago - Ardipithecus Kadabba and Ramidus appear in Ethiopia.

- 4 million years ago - Australopithecus Anamensis appears in East Africa.

- 3.8 to 2.9 million years ago - Australopithecus Afarensis, including the famous fossil "Lucy," found in East Africa

- 2.5 to 1.5 million years ago - Early Homo species, such as Homo Habilis and Homo Rudolfensis, emerge in Africa.

- 1.9 million years ago - Homo Erectus appears, spreading out of Africa into Eurasia and exhibiting more advanced stone tool technology.

- 430,000 years ago - Homosapiens (human) also known as Neanderthal and Caveman emerged in Western Europe.

- 70,000 to 40,000 years ago - Homosapiens (Neanderthal) begin migrating out of Africa, eventually spreading across the globe.

- 6,000 years ago, the Sumerians show up and tell us all about their civilization.

This timeline provides a basic overview of the history of hominoids leading to humans.

I suspect that regardless of how and when human-like animals got here, it is highly likely that we were opportunistic eaters and ate whatever we could. If we were placed in the Garden of Eden, we would enjoy that. If we moved out and had to find other things, we would.

I can guarantee that hominids figured out pretty quickly that "if you don't eat, you die," and so they did the best they could. In the early days, they did not have tools and would have been relegated to eating only plants or whatever 'road kill' they could scavenge.

By excavating ancient sites in Africa, we know that early humans - Homo-erectus was a meat eater dating back to 2.5 million years ago. Animal bones with butchery markings on the bones have been found to indicate Homo erectus did indeed butcher animals.

Pounding bones with stones and bone breakage for dietary and non-dietary reasons are also evident, possibly to get at the marrow inside them or splintering the bone for other reasons.

However, it is impossible to know exactly what they were eating because soft tissue (stomach and digestive tract) does not preserve (for millions of years) to know what was in their systems.

Some of the oldest human artifacts discovered to date are believed to be the Lomekwi 3 stone tools, found in

Kenya, Africa, and dated approximately 3.3 million years ago.

These tools were discovered in 2015 and predate the previously known oldest tools by about 700,000 years. They consist of crude stone flakes and cores, suggesting early hominids were capable of intentional tool-making far earlier than previously thought. These artifacts provide important insights into our early ancestors' cognitive abilities and behaviors.

The exact purpose of the Lomekwi stone tools is still debated among archaeologists and anthropologists. However, based on their characteristics and the context in which they were found, these tools were likely used for various tasks related to processing food and accessing resources.

Some researchers propose that the Lomekwi tools were used for butchering animals, processing plant materials, or pounding and breaking open nuts and seeds. Others suggest they may have been used for digging or scraping tasks.

While the specific function of these tools remains uncertain, their discovery provides important insights into our ancestors' early technological capabilities and adaptive behaviors. They represent a significant milestone in human history, demonstrating early hominids' ability to manipulate and shape their environment using stone tools.

The Lomekwi stone tools do not prove definitively that they ate animals, nor do they prove a strict plant-based diet was consumed. The discovery simply means they were smart and could make tools. The purpose of those tools is yet to be known.

It is important to recognize here that many Jews, Christians, and Muslims believe that the Earth is only 6,000 to 10,000 years old based on genealogies and chronologies found in the Old Testament of the Bible. However, not all Jews, Christians, or Muslims subscribe to the Young Earth theory. Many of them, including those within mainstream denominations, accept scientific evidence supporting an Earth that is billions of years old. They often reconcile their faith with scientific discoveries, interpreting the creation stories in the Bible allegorically rather than literally.

But **this book is not about Religious debate on the age of the Earth**; we are trying to understand what early humans ate and why, so please stay with me here.

The Lomekwi stone tools, found in Kenya (among many other ancient archeological finds), fly in the face of most religious beliefs that the Earth is only a few thousand years old. But without getting into an archaeological or religious debate about how old the Earth is, let's agree that early human civilizations first started in the equatorial regions somewhere around Africa or the Middle East, shall we?

And let's be clear: Just because we find an ancient artifact does not mean that it is the only evidence or the definitive answer to anything. An ancient find is simply that (a discovery); it doesn't necessarily mean or prove anything. Take, for example, the Lomekwi stone tools; even expert archeologists cannot agree on what exactly they were used for.

In Summary,

Our ancient ancestors foraged and hunted, consuming a wide array of plants and animals based on availability and necessity. As hunter-gatherers, greens, nuts, seeds, fruits, and the occasional catch of the day composed the menu. It's amusing when we think about it - our forebears didn't fuss over food blogs or diet trends; they ate what the earth offered and thrived on the nutritional diversity.

However, this changed dramatically with the dawning of agriculture when the Sumerians showed up roughly 4,000 BCE (Before the Common Era). Our ancestors slowly transitioned from nomadic bands to settled communities, planting seeds that blossomed into fields of wheat, barley, and legumes.

It was a pivotal moment that deserves more than a footnote. This **agrarian** (cultivation of land) shift didn't just alter landscapes; it transformed diets. Communities could grow and store food, leading to a steady supply of grains that eventually became staples of the human diet. But while this reliance on grain cultivation enabled human civilizations to flourish, it subtly edged out the broad spectrum of plant foods that had once been the foundation of our nutrition.

The journey to present-day eating habits is fraught with twists and turns. If we peel back the layers of historical diets, we reveal a significant thread - the healthiest patterns are deeply rooted in plant consumption.

History is replete with examples of societies thriving on primarily plant-based diets, enjoying robust health and endurance. It's quite telling that it wasn't the meat-centered feasts of kings and conquerors that held the key to optimum health but rather the simple, plant-rich fare of the common folk. Understanding this could be a game changer, guiding us towards dietary choices that align with our physiology and offering a sustainable path for our health and the environment.

Evolution of Eating Habits

Our journey through the prehistoric buffet line is a fascinating tale of adaptation and survival.

In the earliest chapters of human history (roughly **6-7 million years ago**), our ancestors were opportunistic eaters - gathering plants, nuts, and seeds, complemented by the occasional scavenged leftovers from predators.

It's a diet that might have lacked culinary awards but held the rich diversity our bodies craved. Fast-forward through time to about **2-3 million years ago**, and we see our foraging habits transformed with the discovery of tools. We began to harness the environment in new ways, diversifying our plates even further. With tools, we were able to hunt animals and prepare food more efficiently. However, the majority of our diet was still mainly plant-based - except for colder climates that demanded more of a meat or fish-based diet.

And then, about **one million years ago**, Homo Erectus discovered fire and began using it as a controlled source of heat to stay warm and cook food. Evidence for this finding is the discovery of wood ash traces found at excavation sites. The introduction of fire revolutionized our eating habits and our very biology.

Cooking not only widened our food choices but made nutrients in certain foods more accessible. If you've ever crunched raw broccoli, you'll appreciate the tender magic a little heat can bring. These changes didn't just affect flavor; they allowed for an energy surplus that fueled brain growth. As early humans advanced their technologies with tools and fire, their brains developed by leaps and bounds as well.

As millennia marched on, hunting became more sophisticated, and meat found its way more regularly into the human diet. Interestingly, though, it was never the main event. Our ancestors were picky - they had to be. They favored plants and fresh produce because they were, more often than not, safer and packed with the nutrients essential for survival. Ol' saber-tooth might have been brag-worthy, but the real trophies in terms of nutrition were the fruits, nuts, and veggies they collected.

The next seismic shift came with the dawn of agriculture with the Sumerian civilization about **6,000 years ago**. This period set the scene for an immense change in dietary patterns. Humans went from nomads and scavengers to farmers, and with this, the proportion of plant-based sustenance skyrocketed. Grains, legumes, fruits - these became the sustenance staples that fed civilizations.

Don't get me wrong, through history; meat has had its moments - the gladiators, the knights, Kings, and Queens, they surely indulged. But, it's critical to recognize that these were periods of exception, not the rule. Our bodies thrived on plants, and while meat played a part, it wasn't the keystone of dietary success.

In fact, if you look at old artwork of Kings and Queens from several hundred years ago, you will notice that most of them are depicted as quite fat and sometimes obese. This is because high animal protein diets contribute to that, as I will explain in later chapters.

So, let's talk about why plants are such powerhouses. Their fiber content alone is a marvel; it aids digestion, helps maintain a healthy weight and curbs disease. Couple this with a cavalcade of vitamins, minerals, and antioxidants, and you've got a veritable shield against many a health woe.

Comparatively, meat draws concerns because all of those highly-touted proteins come packaged with saturated fats, cholesterol, and, increasingly, more antibiotics and hormones than you would care to think about.

Modern eating habits have unfortunately shifted away from our ancient plant-loving ways. In early human history, our diet was (on average) about 90% plant-based and 10% animal proteins. In today's world, our diet is almost exactly the opposite: 90% animal proteins and 10% fruits and veggies. Also, massive sugar intake, processed meats, and fast food reign supreme in a world that's forgotten the legacy of leafy greens. It's something that needs addressing because chronic diseases are rising, and our diets are definitely the cause.

The picture painted by history is clear. Humans haven't just survived on a predominantly plant-based diet; they've flourished. Our ancestors plucked their sustenance from the ground and the trees, and it's here that our biological compass points us to what's best for our bodies. The whispers of eons suggest that meat, while capable of sustaining us in moderation, doesn't promise the vibrant health that plants do.

We stand at a crossroads, equipped with knowledge from the past, facing choices that will shape our future and our health. While meat has been a supporting actor in the human dietary drama, the star of the show, the hero in green armor, has been (and should continue to be) plants. It's not just about survival anymore; it's about thriving. If we listen to the echoes of history, leading a life rich in plant-based foods is not just possible; it's the foundation of vitality.

So let's take a leaf from the annals of our ancestors and embrace the botanical bounty that's sustained us for eons. We've evolved not just to endure but to prosper, with plants at the core of our dietary universe. A future that focuses on plant-based eating isn't just paying homage to our past - it's a smart way forward for our health and the health of our planet.

The Shift to Agrarian Societies

As we delve deeper into the histories of the human diet, let's examine a pivotal turn in our **alimentary** (meaning nourishment, pursuit of nutrition, or furnishing sustenance) journey. I am talking about the shift toward an **Agrarian culture** or agricultural society. This transition was more than just a change in food production; it was a revolution in human culture and health.

Before this monumental shift, our hunter-gatherer ancestors roamed the lands at the mercy of nature's offerings. Their diets were diverse, depending on seasonal availability, and heavily reliant on plants. With the advent of agriculture, communities settled down, and for the first time, they had the means to control their food supply. They began to grow their sustenance from the earth, favoring grains like wheat, rice, and corn, which could be stored for long periods and supported growing populations.

This change, which occurred about 10,000 to 6,000 years ago, was not just a logistical step towards civilization; it also marked a profound difference in humans' diets from varied and plant-rich to more grain-centered. Over time, as agricultural societies developed, so did the cultivation of plants and domesticated animals - but with an unintended consequence. Plants were increasingly sidelined on the plate as animal husbandry grew more sophisticated and meat more abundant.

Interestingly, however, the initially plant-heavy diets of these early farmers tell us something about our dietary needs. These populations thrived on diets rich in vegetables, fruits, legumes, and whole grains - the staples we now know lower the risk of chronic diseases and support overall health. These whole foods, provided by the earth, were the building blocks of human health and fueled the daily lives of our ancestors.

The predominance of plant-based nutrition in early agricultural societies also illustrates the sustainability of this diet. While raising animals for consumption began to take hold, it wasn't until much later that meat consumption at today's levels became possible - or thinkable. Why? Because raising animals for food requires vast amounts of resources, including land, water, and crops, to feed them, making it an inefficient use of resources compared to plant cultivation.

Moreover, looking back, it's clear that meat was not the everyday fare but rather a luxury for many. Regular consumption of animal products was historically reserved for the affluent, while the less fortunate relied on what the earth naturally provided. This disparity highlighted a socio-economic and nutritional divide that would later have health implications as diets rich in animal fats became more commonplace with increased wealth and industrialization.

Now, why does this matter to us in our current dietary context? As we consider moving toward plant-based diets, we are not embarking on a newfangled trend but returning to our roots. With its initial heavy reliance on plants, the shift to agricultural societies shows us that a plant-based diet isn't just sustainable; it agrees with the blueprint of human health and social development.

As we consider the modern health crises of obesity, heart disease, and diabetes, it's hard not to acknowledge that a diet high in animal products has not served us well in terms of health outcomes. It takes us away from our agrarian ancestors' nutrient-dense, high-fiber diets towards a path riddled with health risks.

Finally, embracing a plant-based diet is a nod to those simpler times when food was grown from the soil, and our plates were teeming with the rich variety of nature's bounty. The burgeoning grain fields of early agrarian societies were a testament to the power of plant nutrition - a lesson that carries profound relevance for our times.

So, we have to wonder, why stray from a diet that saw our ancestors through the dawn of civilization? It seems like it's time to shift back, don't you think?

Chapter 2: Carnivore vs. Herbivore - Anatomy Tells a Story

When you dive into the anatomical structures of carnivores compared to herbivores, nature reveals clues as to what each creature is naturally designed to eat.

- carnivores are optimized for predation

- Herbivores are optimized for foraging

- All animals must procure their food in an energy efficient manner

Carnivorous animals are optimized for predation: They are built for the hunt. They have light-weight limbs designed to run fast with long, sharp claws and teeth to catch and kill prey.

Animals designed to eat other animals must run fast with weapons to overcome and subdue their prey because their food doesn't want to be eaten. Even though carnivores can run fast, they do not have the endurance a plant eater has.

Herbivores (like humans) have big, heavy feet and thick, heavy legs (that require a lot of energy to run), unlike carnivores, who have thin legs and tiny feet that require less energy to move.

When we look at a true carnivore like a wolf or cheetah, we see that they are built for speed, very fast, and their vulnerable parts (stomach and reproductive organs) are protected in the back. They have thick, strong muscle and bone around the neck and shoulder area for padding so that when they are kicked by an animal that doesn't want to be eaten, they are not injured.

We will talk more about their teeth, skeletal, and digestive systems, but let's talk about herbivores for a moment.

Herbivores are optimized for foraging

Herbivores have sharp teeth in the front for cutting, flat molars in the back designed for grinding fibrous plant materials, and a jaw that can move side to side for effective chewing - not slicing or tearing. But teeth tell just half the tale because the real magic happens in the digestive system.

Carnivores have a simple, short gut, allowing for rapid digestion of protein and fat before it begins to rot. Herbivores (and humans) feature a longer, more complex digestive system with plenty of twists and turns, ideal for the slow and steady breakdown of plant fibers and nutrients.

An herbivore's digestive system is designed to slowly unravel the complex structures of plants, extracting every last nutrient it can, but more on this later.

All animals must procure their food energy-efficiently, or they will go extinct.

If an animal has to constantly expend more energy trying to procure its food than it gains from eating its food, it will only survive for a short time. So, animals that consume plants are designed to forage over great distances and spend little energy acquiring food.

You don't need to be an anthropologist to know that an animal's anatomy tells a story, but let's take a closer look at skeletal systems to see if we can figure out the difference between herbivores and carnivores.

The Skeletal Contrast

Let's lean in and examine the intricate story our skeletons tell about our dietary heritage. It's fascinating how much you can deduce from an animal's eating habits by paying close attention to their bones.

It's like piecing together a millennia-old puzzle, one that can enlighten our modern-day food choices and, spoiler alert, it nudges us gently towards those leafy greens.

Carnivores, for example, have robust skeletal structures that support their ambush and pursuit lifestyles. Their bones are designed to endure the stress of a kill, with powerful joints for swift, spring-loaded action. A carnivore's spine is spring-loaded for power and ready to pounce.

Think about how the skeletal systems of carnivores seem to bolster their predatory lifestyle:

- Heavy, muscular necks and jaws.

- Shoulders that can withstand a punch (or rather a kick).

- Tails that balance out their ferocious sprints.

Regarding their skeletal structure, carnivores, like dogs, cats, wolves, etc., have a **digitigrade** stance, meaning they are permanently up on their toes. In other words, they are designed in a permanent "runner's crouch" position where it costs energy just to stand or walk because their muscles must resist gravity to stay on all fours.

Herbivores have either an unguligrade or plantigrade stance. An **unguligrade** stance means the animal literally stands on its toenails or hoofs like the horse or pig, while a **plantigrade** stance means the animal walks or stands on its whole foot like a human or bear.

Side note: Although humans and bears are classified as omnivores, it might surprise you that a bear's diet is 90% plant matter and 10% other animals that they scavenge.

One more comment on stance: In the wild, primates have a semi-plantigrade stance (with the heel elevated), while the chimpanzee (our closest primate relative) also has a plantigrade stance.

And speaking of feet, primates lack those razor-sharp claws made for tearing into flesh, and instead, we have toes suitable for balance and prolonged bipedal locomotion. Once again, our bodies seem primed for picking apples rather than ambushing antelopes.

The skeleton of an herbivore isn't interested in a sudden pounce either; instead, it's constructed for the long haul - literally. The structure of a herbivore has the stamina for extensive migration and the constant meanderings of grazing.

The leg bones showcase less about brute force and more about the endurance needed to roam vast distances in search of fresh pastures.

So, where do we humans fit into this skeletal narrative? If we were to put ourselves under the same scrutiny, human bones and bodies aren't made to withstand the rigors of taking down prey.

Some of us might be tough enough to play American football or Rugby for a couple of hours, but if all of us had to do that day in and day out, all day long, to catch our meals, we would have gone extinct a long time ago.

We lack those telltale signs of a carnivorous predator - our skeletons are closer to those lengthy striders you find nibbling on shrubbery. Our bones suggest patience, endurance, and a rather un-carnivorous lack of speed typically required to chase down our dinner.

One interesting fact about herbivores (in contrast to carnivores) is that herbivores are designed with their center of mass directly over their pillars or legs. As mentioned above, carnivores must use muscle energy to stand up, whereas herbivores use very little energy to stand. Indeed, walking for a human is a form of graceful, controlled falling where gravity does most of the work, and we spend very little energy walking.

An herbivore's weight is positioned directly over its limbs so that gravity is resisted by the animal's skeletal system, not muscle. Some herbivores spend so little energy to stand that they can actually sleep while standing.

Our upright spines testify to our posture and ability to walk well for long distances. They cradle our center of gravity and give us that upright advantage, freeing our hands for foraging rather than ferocious hunting.

Our hip and thigh bones are weight-bearing marvels that indicate our ancestors might've had more success strolling through the prehistoric grocery aisles than sprinting after nimble and fast prey.

Chew on this: Our jaws are remarkably less robust than typical carnivores. As you will discover in a moment, the average carnivore has a 5 to 10 times stronger bite than a human's.

Our jaw's hinge and muscle structure, with our rather pedestrian-looking teeth, hardly scream predator. We're built for a menu more about grinding and masticating plant fibers rather than shredding cartilage and bone.

Understanding our anatomy can help steer us toward a diet more aligned with what our bodies have been shaped to handle across the eons. It becomes clear that our bones sing a sonnet of berries and fruit without the need for claws and fangs. Our biology is nudging toward a plate brimming with plants.

As we close the chapter on our skeletal system, let's carry forward this understanding to inform our choices at the dining table. Our bones have a story to tell that champions a life sustained by the bountiful garden rather than the hunt. By aligning our diet with the blueprint provided by our anatomy, we're not just paying homage to our lineage but also investing in a future where our health blooms in the most natural, plant-powered way.

Carnivore Predation vs. Herbivore Mobility

The animal kingdom has evolved various survival strategies, and two of the most significant are the distinction between carnivore predation and a herbivore's mobility for foraging. These are profound insights into the understanding of diet and how it shapes the very fabric of nature, including our health and well-being.

Please note: There is a lot of overlap in this section because I need to recap some core issues to expand on them as well as drive the points home, so please indulge me if it sounds like I am repeating a few things we just talked about in the previous section.

And besides, I'm hoping you might retain some of this better if I say it a few times in different ways :-)

Carnivore Predation

Carnivores are equipped with powerful, lightweight legs for running fast. Their sharp claws and teeth are designed for tearing flesh and are the epitome of predation. Their bodies are made to catch, kill, and consume other animals. Speed is often their ally, but it's the short, intense sprints they're adapted for, not endurance. They must overpower their prey quickly or risk losing out on a meal.

Therefore, they need to be intelligent and cunning so they don't waste much energy trying to catch their meal. Carnivores do not go after the biggest or strongest; they seek out the weak, the old, the young, the diseased, or the injured because they are the easiest to catch.

Their senses are finely tuned to hearing, smelling, and finding other animals. Their ears, for example, can move around to help find the direction of other animals or prey. Their sense of smell is many magnitudes stronger than that of an herbivore. Carnivores can smell infections and even cancer or metabolic disorders in other animals from a distance. This is how they know which ones to go after and not waste a lot of energy trying to catch the healthy ones.

Because of this predatory skill set, they strengthen the prey species' gene pool by eliminating the weak, diseased, old, or stupid ones.

Carnivores are scavengers and will eat dead or dying animals. They are Mother Nature's cleanup crew and have the digestive system to handle rotting or diseased flesh. Carnivores have a physiology that allows them to eat rotting tissue, but herbivores do not. The energy content from a rotting carcass is the same as that of a freshly killed one.

Herbivores and humans, however, have an instinct to repulse at the idea of eating a rotting carcass, while a carnivore would eat and enjoy it.

In stark contrast to carnivores, herbivores don't want the sick or the diseased; they desire the most healthy, beautiful, vibrant, lush vegetation because it is the most nutrient-dense. An herbivore is not a scavenger and will not eat dead or dying plants or animals.

Predation with an herbivore mentality is destructive because it drives the extinction of the prey species by going after the strongest, the best, the most vibrant, or healthy animals. When modern humans hunt, they go after the strongest, biggest, most beautiful, and most healthy animals, which is extremely harmful to the gene pool of the animals we hunt.

Herbivore Mobility & Mindset

Humans and many herbivores have heavy feet (unlike carnivores built for speed) and a plantigrade stance. Plantigrade (as mentioned earlier) refers to a type of locomotion or stance in which an animal walks with its entire foot flat on the ground. This is in contrast to digitigrade (carnivores walking on toes) and unguligrade (certain other herbivores that walk on their hooves) locomotion.

In plantigrade animals (such as humans, bears, and raccoons), the heel and sole of the foot make contact with the ground during walking or running. This type of locomotion typically provides stability and weight distribution across the entire foot, allowing for more flexibility in movement and a greater ability to navigate various terrain.

Before you tell me that bears and raccoons are carnivores, let me say that bears and raccoons are omnivores. While some bear species, such as the giant panda, are primarily herbivorous and feed mainly on bamboo or plant material, most are omnivorous. Omnivorous bears, like the grizzly bear and black bear, have a diet of various foods, including vegetation such as berries, roots, grasses, insects, fish, small mammals, and carrion (dead animals).

Raccoons are opportunistic feeders with a diverse diet that eat a wide range of foods depending on availability and season, including fruits, nuts, seeds, insects, and small animals like rodents, amphibians, and bird eggs.

Overall, bears and raccoons exhibit omnivorous feeding behavior, consuming plant and animal-based foods to meet their nutritional needs, but let's not get too far down the rabbit hole here. I am clarifying that they are omnivores, not carnivores.

Getting back to energy conservation and the cost of locomotion or mobility, all animals must procure their food energy efficiently. Humans are designed to walk to forage, not run down an animal to kill it.

Endurance

Herbivores rely on endurance. Their bodies are designed to travel long distances for foraging. The plants that an herbivore wants to eat are usually spread out, and they must travel to get enough food. They are designed with straight limbs supporting their body mass in a way that requires little energy to stand or walk. Many herbivores can sleep while standing.

Humans have an upright stance because it is an extremely efficient position for foraging. We can run (not as fast as carnivores), but we are much better walkers. In fact, when a human walks, it is actually a form of controlled falling, which costs very little energy to walk.

Herbivores can typically run for much longer distances at a steady pace, and this isn't by chance or accident. Herbivores are designed to graze and roam across vast terrains in search of vegetation. Their key to survival isn't in the fight but in the flight. Their legs can carry them long distances but are also capable of agile movements to escape predators. It's a dance of life and death, powered by legs designed for different tunes.

Herbivores tend to be active during the day when carnivores are asleep, while most carnivores have better night vision and hunt at night when herbivores are asleep. Herbivores tend to live longer than carnivores due to the higher intake of antioxidants.

Why does this matter to a human diet? Let's look at the bigger picture: The agility and endurance of herbivores have allowed them to thrive on a diet composed exclusively of plants. They're proof that you can not only survive but flourish with a lifestyle that avoids the consumption of animal flesh.

Regarding humans specifically, we were never the fastest runners in the savannah, nor did we possess the raw power of a predator. Yet we have survived and thrived, not because of our physical prowess, but because of our wit, ability to cooperate, and adaptability, including dietary flexibility.

Omnivores

It is true that humans are Omnivores, but just because we can tolerate and consume meat (in moderate proportions) doesn't mean it's optimal or that we should. Our bodies aren't designed for the rapid digestion and assimilation of flesh like carnivores.

On examining the characteristics of herbivorous creatures further, we find that they have the mobility for ongoing travel and the digestive systems to take in a wide variety of foliage. This intake of plants provides them with complex carbohydrates, fibers, and a host of essential vitamins and minerals - components largely absent from a carnivorous diet.

Human beings are unique and have survived as omnivores. This point isn't disputed, but we're reaching a moment in time where we have to ask ourselves what's sustainable **for our bodies and the environment**.

Shifting away from meat and toward a plant-rich diet acknowledges the natural endurance and health benefits that herbivores experience alongside their mobility, endurance, and ability to forage.

Consider the link between a plant-based diet and improved cardiovascular health. Just as herbivores benefit from their high-fiber diet to move swiftly over large terrains, humans may experience better blood flow and stamina due to the heart-healthy effects of plant nutrients.

Meat, on the other hand, especially red and processed meat, has been linked with numerous health concerns such as heart disease and stroke, topics we'll explore in later sections.

Finally, let's talk about the energy aspect. You don't need massive bursts of energy to tackle a broccoli spear. But you do need sustained energy to fuel your day. Unlike meat products, plants are replete with complex carbohydrates that are nature's battery to release energy slowly over time.

Even though we may not need to outrun predators, our modern-day challenges demand endurance, focus, and long-term health that a plant-based diet is known to support.

Migrating to a plant-based diet is a positive herbivore strategy to emphasize long-term health, harmony with nature, and a sustainable future. Going Vegan (or at least Vegetarian) is a profound step that respects the natural order and acknowledges our true capabilities (that we're built not for chasing down prey) but for gathering nature's bounty.

Constantly on the move, covering life's distances with persistent grace, we're much like herbivores, finding sustenance and power in plants.

Dentition and Digestion

Have you ever looked at your teeth in the mirror and wondered about the significance of their varied shapes?

Those incisors, canines, molars, and their placement aren't just random; they tell an evolutionary tale of diet and digestion.

Like lions and tigers, Carnivores are equipped with large, sharp fangs designed for seizing and tearing flesh. Their digestive tracts are short, highly acidic, and efficient at breaking down protein and fat. This makes sense for animals whose diets are primarily meat-based.

On the other hand, herbivores boast a different dental design tailored for plant consumption. The flat molars humans have at the back of our mouths are perfect for grinding foliage and fibrous plants.

Rather than carnivores' short, simple digestive tracts, herbivores have longer and more complex system designed to extract all the goodness from high-fiber diets. They host a variety of bacteria in their guts that help break down cellulose, an ability truly foreign to natural meat-eaters. The reason for a shorter digestive tract in a carnivore is that most of the digestion and assimilation is done in the stomach with a very high acid composition.

Once the meat, bone, cartilage, and fur have been assimilated (as well as they're going to be), the remains need to get out of the body quickly so they don't rot or putrefy in the animal.

In contrast, an herbivore has a much longer digestive system (relative to size). The digestive system of a 300 pound cat is roughly 15 feet, while the digestive tract of a human is about 25-30 feet. Obese humans that weigh 300-500 lbs still have the same 25-30 foot digestive system.

While cats and humans have digestive systems adapted to their respective dietary habits, humans generally have longer digestive tracts due to the additional structures involved in processing plant-based foods and extracting nutrients from a wider range of sources. Plant matter like cellulose or fiber must stay in the tract longer for the nutrients to be absorbed. If meat is allowed to stay in a longer digestive system for a longer period, it can rot and putrefy in there and create a whole lot of other mischief.

Where does that place us, though? Our teeth are a mixed bag. Those canines of ours might seem like proof of carnivorous intent, but they pale in comparison to the fangs of actual predators. Our molars and premolars are flat, perfect for grinding grains and vegetables. Our digestive tracts are more akin to herbivores: longer than carnivores' and including a microbiome that thrives on fiber.

Imagine, if you will, the digestion process from a mechanical standpoint. Eating plants typically require more chewing, is a less violent, and a more methodical process that starts the digestive process off on the right foot, or tooth, as it were. This extra effort, this thorough grinding, facilitates a more efficient breakdown once the food reaches the stomach and intestines.

The prevailing wisdom in nutrition circles points out that a more extended digestive process, like that required for plant matter, supports a slower and steadier release of nutrients into our bloodstream.

This prevents the notorious sugar spikes associated with high-glycemic meals, often comprising processed foods. Stability in blood sugar is a coveted attribute in managing weight and preventing diabetes, highlighting yet another feather in the cap of a plant-based diet.

And let's talk about fiber, shall we? Fiber is a plant-based nutrient (absent in meat) that performs wonders for our digestion. Fiber aids in pulling toxins out of our body regulates bowel movements and has a role in maintaining healthy cholesterol levels. Interestingly, fiber also helps us feel full longer, promoting weight management without the need for calorie counting or unnaturally restrictive diets.

While easing into a discussion on bowel health might make some squirm, it's imperative to understand that the regularity and quality of our bowel movements are crucial indicators of our overall well-being. Plant-rich diets lead to healthier, more consistent bathroom visits - something that can't be said for a diet heavy in meat, which can strain our digestive systems.

The stark differences in the digestion and absorption of nutrients between carnivores and herbivores hint at what is natural for us. While some argue that we are not strict herbivores, our bodies undeniably lean towards that design.

Sure, we have the means to digest meat (in moderation), but it's far from our most efficient fuel. It comes down to whether you'd prefer your body to operate like a well-oiled machine or one that's overburdened and struggling to cope with demands outside its design specifications.

So, as we chew on the facts of dentition and digestion, it becomes progressively clear that a plant-based diet aligns more closely with our anatomy.

Change can be challenging, but it's comforting to realize that our bodies have been whispering (or perhaps, through the rumble of indigestion, shouting) their preference for a plant-centered diet all along. It's not about adapting to something new but returning to what our bodies know best.

Understanding our anatomical predisposition for a plant-based diet isn't just food for thought; it's the very essence of building our meals and our health. With each plant-based choice, we're not just eating; we're honoring the natural design of our bodies. And in doing so, we promote a more vibrant, energetic, and disease-resistant self.

Fangs Against Flatness

While we've ventured far from our ancestral roots, our teeth remain a blueprint of our intended diet - one without the sharp fangs typically associated with ripping through tough flesh.

As we've explored before, human teeth, much like those of herbivores, are designed for grinding and mashing rather than the slashing and shearing actions perfected by carnivores.

Mouth, Teeth & Jaw

Looking at the mouth, we see a huge contrast between herbivores and carnivores.

Investigating the business end of a carnivore reveals an eating machine, while the mouth of an herbivore closely resembles what humans have been endowed with. And while some humans can also be considered "an eating machine," I'm talking about teeth here, not how much they eat.

Carnivores boast impressive fangs and sharp, jagged molars designed to slice and tear flesh, while herbivores have sharp teeth in the front for cutting but flat molars in the back for grinding and pulverizing.

The jaw structure is also different. Carnivores' jaw hinges like scissors for cutting, while herbivores have an "L-shaped" jaw that is more like a nutcracker for grinding. A carnivore's jaw can only move up and down in a scissor motion, while an herbivore's jaw can move up and down and side to side for chewing and grinding. By the way, carnivores generally do not chew their food;

they bite off manageable chunks and swallow whole pieces of flesh.

So if you've ever wondered why your dog seems to woof down his or her food without chewing, now you know why.

Carnivores have a powerful bite that can produce 500 to 1,000 pounds per square inch of pressure, whereas humans can only create about 150-200 psi of bite pressure. So think about that the next time you want to consider running down a rabbit and biting a chunk of its hide, fur, and flesh.

I know what you're thinking, "But wait, we have 'canine teeth' !?" No, we don't. Canine means dog, and we are not dogs; dogs are carnivores. What we have are called incisors and bicuspid (pre-molar) teeth. It is true that incisors and bicuspids are there for biting or cutting, but they were designed for apples, not tearing the flesh from an animal.

Calling that pointy tooth in our mouth a canine tooth is ignorant and misleading, fooling people into thinking they are carnivores.

Our "canine teeth" simply aren't comparable to the pronounced fangs of actual predators or carnivores. Ours are more subdued and far less lethal, speaking to a diet based more on plants than the predatory practices of our mammalian cousins.

So, what happens when our diet consists of heavy meat consumption despite our flat, herbivore-leaning dentition?

Well, it's like using a butter knife when the job calls for a steak knife - it doesn't quite work. Our jaws are designed for chewing fibrous plant materials, nuts, seeds, and legumes. This aligns much better with our dental anatomy, promoting better digestion and overall health from the beginning of the digestive process.

Consider also the impact on your pearly whites. Teeth bathed in the nutrients of a plant-based diet tend to fare better in terms of dental health - less exposure to the acids and bacterial promotion that come with meat-based diets.

On the other hand, when we fuel our bodies with the naturally water-rich and fibrous bounty of plants, we're nourishing ourselves and "brushing" our teeth with every bite of crunchy vegetables and fruits. It's a win-win that starts with a smile.

Moreover, think about the struggle our teeth go through when chomping on meat. The effort required to break down animal flesh is far from the design our teeth suggest.

It's a mismatch that can lead to excessive wear, dental problems, and even jaw issues over time. By opting for cuisine our teeth can handle more efficiently, we cater to our anatomical strengths and reduce risks associated with physical dental trauma caused by inappropriate diets.

And it's not only about the mechanical aspects but also the chemistry. A plant-based diet provides an alkaline environment that supports tooth enamel health, whereas the acidity from a meat-centered diet may promote decay and weaken enamel over time.

Eating animal products is very acidic, so eating your greens could mean fewer cavities and less dental erosion, emphasizing the notion that our diets should reflect our design for a host of benefits.

So you're saying that our lack of fangs and molars that cut (in contrast to ones that grind), this points to a natural inclination towards plant consumption? Absolutely.

Not because we can't occasionally indulge in other food items but because our anatomy sings the praises of a plant-based diet in a chorus as old as humankind itself. It's a melody of wellness that plays out in more ways than just dental health.

Another consideration is the digestion process itself. It begins in the mouth, where enzymes in saliva start to break down food.

While carnivores have saliva meant to clamp down and kill bacteria in meat, ours is best equipped to initiate the breakdown of carbohydrates found in plant foods. This subtle nuance in saliva makeup hints once again at the evolutionary pathways that have favored a diet built around plants.

Dare to consider the implications for your own meals - a dietary plan that respects the blueprints nature has given us. Embracing plants in our daily consumption isn't just about preventing lifestyle diseases or controlling weight; it's also about honoring the structure and function of our bodies as they've been designed.

When you crunch into that next piece of raw carrot or that crisp apple, remember that you're doing exactly what your teeth were meant to do.

So, toss aside the myth that humans are natural-born carnivores. We possess no killer instincts or hunting prowess manifested in our dental anatomy. Our so-called "fangs" are a far cry from the lethal weapons seen in our carnivorous counterparts. Instead, they're perfectly designed for an abundant variety of plant foods that can lead us to optimal health.

In summary, our teeth aren't just there for the smiles; they're our quiet advocates for a plant-based diet. They implore us to reconsider and align our eating habits with their humble structure.

It's time we listen to our bodies, a fundamental principle ignored far too often in the debate over our dietary destinies. Let's allow nature's design to guide us back to a diet that's as flat, wide, and beautifully diverse as our teeth.

Chapter 3: The Myth of Meat - Busting Protein Misconceptions

A towering myth hovers over dinner tables and gym conversations: the idea that meat is the ultimate source of protein.

In this chapter, we will dismantle this urban legend for good. Many of us grew up with the mantra that meat equals muscle, as if cows, pigs, and chickens monopolize the protein market. But consider this: The strongest animals on the planet, like elephants and gorillas, build their mighty physiques on greens. Could it be that spinach and kale might be the true heavyweights in the protein world?

It's time to dig into the meat of the matter and look at protein quality and sources. You might have been led to believe that only animal-based foods can provide 'complete' proteins with all the essential amino acids your body craves.

But, spoiler alert: **plants have all the amino acids you need**! In fact, by combining different plant-based foods throughout the day, you get a symphony of nutrients working in perfect harmony. No meat necessary. As for quality, plant proteins are like a breath of fresh air to your cells compared to their meaty counterparts.

They come packaged with fiber and antioxidants, and none of the baggage animal proteins carry, like cholesterol and saturated fats.

Aside from quality, there's the persistent myth of incomplete plant proteins, which we'll obliterate once and for all. 'Incomplete' is a term that's been misleadingly slapped onto plant proteins for too long.

Every plant contains all nine essential amino acids, albeit in different ratios. Unless you're munching on one specific plant all day, you're likely getting a complete protein profile.

It's all about mixing and matching: Beans with rice, peanut butter on whole-grain toast, or a colorful veggie stir-fry. By diversifying your plant intake, you're not just squashing this incomplete protein myth: You're investing in a diverse portfolio of nutrients that can pay off with incredible health dividends.

Protein Quality and Sources

When it comes to protein, many folks still hold onto the idea that meat is the end-all, be-all source of this vital macronutrient. But let's set things straight: protein quality isn't determined by animal origin. The notion that plant proteins are somehow inferior is one of those myths that's ripe for debunking. You will be surprised to learn that a world of protein-rich possibilities lies beyond the meat aisle.

First, let's talk about what makes a protein "high quality." Amino acids are the building blocks of protein. Our bodies need a set of 20 different amino acids, 9 of which are considered "essential," but we cannot make them ourselves (we have to get them from our diets).

In other words, animals cannot synthesize all of the amino acids needed for protein synthesis and other essential physiological functions. These amino acids, known as essential amino acids, must be obtained from the animal's diet.

Essential amino acids can be incredibly easy to get over the course of a day by eating a variety of typical food combinations such as rice and beans, hummus and pita, or peanut butter on whole wheat bread (these classic combos are not just tasty, they're incredibly protein-savvy, too.)

It's also helpful to realize that your body is incredibly smart. It recycles amino acids to form complete proteins all on its own. You don't need to meticulously plan every meal to ensure you're getting every essential amino acid every time. Nature and your body's biology have got your back.

Moreover, by looking beyond meat for protein, you'll stumble upon many nutritional bonuses. Plant proteins bring fiber, antioxidants, and a spectrum of vitamins and minerals that meat can't boast. These extra players are fundamental in the symphony that is our overall health; they reduce inflammation, bolster our immune system, and support our digestive health.

Let's face it: we live in a society that's overly fixated on meat and protein intake, often pushing consumption far beyond our actual requirements.

The truth is, as long as you're consuming enough calories, it's pretty hard not to get enough protein, even on a plant-based diet. And rest assured, the protein in these plants is of stellar quality, allowing your body to thrive, repair, and grow.

Consider the diversity available in plant-based protein sources. Leafy greens like spinach and kale, legumes like lentils, chickpeas, and black beans. Also, grains such as farro and teff; nuts like almonds and walnuts; seeds such as hemp, flax, and pumpkin. The list goes on and is deliciously extensive. This variety is good for your taste buds and body, providing a broad arsenal of amino acids while keeping your meals exciting.

If you're worried about bulking up and building muscle, relax. Plant power has you covered there, too. A multitude of vegan athletes are now thriving on plant-based diets, cashing in on the dense nutrition profile without the extra baggage that often comes with animal proteins, like unhealthy fats and cholesterol.

I'll level with you – it's easy to fall victim to the "where do you get your protein" paranoia that's been peddled for decades. But knowledge and educating yourself about this can be powerful.

With the correct information, we can all make better nutritional choices. Embracing plant-based proteins isn't just a viable option; it's a pathway to a healthier life filled with nutrient-dense, sustainable, and ethical food choices that promote well-being for ourselves and the planet.

So next time you wonder, "Where can I get my protein?" you might want to skip the steak and reach for a black bean burger instead. Trust me, your body (and the planet) will thank you. Transitioning to plant-based proteins isn't that difficult, and it can also be an adventure in flavor and nutrition that supports your health in ways that meat simply can't match.

The Myth of Incomplete Plant Proteins

Leaning into the heart of the protein myth, let's tackle a common misconception that's been wilting the reputation of plant-based diets for years. The notion that plant proteins are inherently 'incomplete' is a myth as persistent as it is inaccurate. It's time to set the record straight once and for all.

Protein & Amino Acids from Plants

First of all, proteins are made of amino acids. Out of 20 different amino acids, our bodies can naturally produce 11. The remaining nine essential amino acids must come from our diet. The myth clings to the idea that only animal-based foods provide all nine. But don't be fooled into thinking that's the only way to protein paradise.

Plants and animals both produce amino acids. Amino acids are the building blocks of proteins, essential for the growth and development of all organisms, including plants and animals. Through photosynthesis, plants produce carbohydrates, which serve as the primary energy source for synthesizing organic molecules, including amino acids.

Plants are capable of synthesizing all of the 20 standard amino acids needed for protein synthesis. They can produce these amino acids through various metabolic pathways, including the conversion of simple molecules such as sugars and nitrogen compounds into amino acids.

Additionally, some amino acids can be obtained by plants through nitrogen uptake from the soil in the form of nitrates or ammonium ions. Plants can then incorporate these nitrogen compounds into amino acids through nitrogen assimilation pathways.

Overall, plants can produce amino acids through internal biosynthetic processes and nitrogen uptake from their environment. These amino acids are essential for synthesizing proteins and other physiological processes within the plant.

Plants, my friends, are hardly the underdogs of the amino acid game. **Virtually all plants contain all nine essential amino acids** in varying ratios.

While it's true that some plant foods are lower in certain amino acids, this isn't the nutrition crisis it's often made out to be. The beauty of a varied plant-based diet is that what one plant lacks, another provides. By eating a spectrum of plant foods, you'll weave a complete amino acid tapestry over the course of the day.

Protein & Amino Acids from Animals

As mentioned above, amino acids are the building blocks of proteins essential for the growth, development, and maintenance of all animal tissues. Animals require amino acids for various physiological processes, including muscle building, hormone synthesis, enzyme, and immune system function.

Animals can produce some amino acids within their bodies through biosynthetic pathways. These amino acids are known as **non-essential** amino acids because they can be synthesized by the animal's cells from other molecules. Examples of non-essential amino acids synthesized by animals include alanine, glutamine, and glycine.

However, **animals cannot synthesize all the amino acids needed for protein synthesis** and other essential physiological functions. These amino acids, known as essential amino acids, **must be obtained from the animal's diet**.

There are nine essential amino acids for humans: histidine, isoleucine, leucine, lysine, methionine, phenylalanine, threonine, tryptophan, and valine. **Animals must consume foods containing these essential amino acids to ensure proper growth, development, and overall health.**

In short, animals synthesize some amino acids within their bodies and obtain others from their diet to meet their nutritional requirements and support essential physiological functions.

"Where do you get your protein?"

Consider that ignorant question busted. The myth that you can only get protein from eating animals is wrong and naive.

Think about it like this: historically, our ancestors didn't have the luxury of nibbling on a single food type all day. Diversity was their survival tactic, and it worked beautifully.

Quinoa, buckwheat, soy, and chia seeds, for instance, are all plant foods that are dazzlingly complete in the amino acid department. But even without these so-called 'complete' proteins at every meal, our bodies are masterful at pooling amino acids from different sources to build complete proteins as needed. There's no need to meticulously combine foods at each meal, a popular concept now discredited by modern nutrition science.

Muscle Building Myths - Busted

Now, let's talk about muscle building and maintenance. It's a common worry that without a steak or chicken breast on your plate, your muscles might just wither away – not so. Plant-based eaters, from weekend warriors to elite athletes, can and do build robust, high-performing muscles. The quality of your overall diet, not just the source of protein, plays a pivotal role in muscle health.

In fact, some of the strongest animals in the wild (like the gorilla, elephant, and rhinoceros) are herbivores. So, to think that you must only eat meat to build strong muscles is ignorant and foolish.

Moreover, while focusing on protein, let's pay attention to the ensemble cast of nutrients that come along for the ride with plant proteins. These tag-alongs include dietary fiber, vitamins, minerals, and phytonutrients that work in concert to support a thriving body. The animal protein package, by contrast, often brings along less-helpful co-stars like saturated fat and cholesterol.

It's time we embrace the dance of plant proteins in our diets, where a legume here and a grain there create a beautiful, complete protein ballet. The myth of incomplete plant proteins stems from outdated studies and misinformation that have sadly overstayed their welcome in our dietary dialogue.

And let's dispel another myth, "you cannot get enough protein from plants." This lie shrinks when you realize that the average person typically consumes far more protein than is necessary.

Have you ever heard of anyone being diagnosed with protein deficiency? It's exceptionally rare in regions where caloric needs are met. Most of us are getting plenty of protein without even trying.

Embracing plants for their protein potential isn't just about bikinis or biceps: It's about nurturing your body from the inside out. When you base your diet around whole, plant-based foods, you are meeting your protein needs and empowering your health on every level while keeping that amino acid or protein myth in the fiction section where it belongs.

So, give peas a chance and let the lentils into your life. Heap your plates with chickpeas, seeds, nuts, tempeh, and all the vibrant veggies you can get your hands on. By doing so, you're investing in your body's critical infrastructure and bankrolling a future of health that's resilient, robust, and ready to enjoy the life you want to lead. Start now and realize a plant-based lifestyle with no myths or compromises, just good, wholesome food that fully satisfies our protein requirements.

The Dark Side of Meat Consumption

Diving deeper into our discussion about meat, it's time to shed light on a concern that's too significant to ignore: the repercussions of meat consumption on our health. The SAD (Standard American Diet) is brimming with meat at every meal, and this lifestyle is mostly to blame for some pretty dire health issues.

Heart disease, heart attacks, strokes, and certain types of diabetes are conditions that lead to discomfort and human lives cut short. There's a giant flashing arrow pointing at the high amounts of saturated fats and cholesterol (typically found in meat consumption) as the culprit. Clogged arteries and meat-heavy diets have been linked with higher blood pressure and high cholesterol levels, Both notorious risk factors for cardiovascular disease.

It makes me SAD to think about all that and how we Americans are killing ourselves with what we put in our bodies.

Diabetes is a lifestyle disease that has been exploding in America at an alarming rate. One big lie we have all been told is that "type 2 diabetes is caused by eating too much sugar or not getting enough exercise". While those things contribute, they are not the cause, and the role of meat consumption has been completely ignored by "experts" and health professionals.

For instance, the high iron content in red meat is associated with an increased risk of type 2 diabetes. The excess cholesterol from eating animals can clog up arteries and block sugar receptor sites in the vascular system, leading to a problem with the body's ability to regulate insulin, which is another issue.

Processed meats are particularly villainous, often full of additives, preservatives, hormones, and steroids that no lab coat professional (with a moral compass) would recommend for healthy consumption. Each bite of that processed meat product could nudge your body's insulin balance off-kilter, setting the stage for diabetes to waltz in.

As we cross that bridge into considering other health risks, let's remember the myriad of diseases that meat consumption can cause or be attributed to. From certain types of cancer to autoimmune diseases, meat's fingerprints are often at the crime scene.

It's like a tangled web wherein each thread connects to another health issue. But fear not; we will expose these issues and arm you with knowledge to empower you to make informed decisions that could lead to a healthier life.

Links to Heart Disease and Stroke

Let's dive right into the heart of the matter - quite literally. Decades of research have drawn a pretty unsettling connection between meat consumption and an increased risk for heart disease and stroke. When you think about it, these two conditions are among the top culprits responsible for premature death and disability.

So, how does meat play into this? First, most meat products are loaded with saturated fats and cholesterol, which are notorious for clogging up arteries. The more clogged your arteries are, the harder it is for blood to flow, setting the stage for heart disease and strokes.

If veins and arteries in and around your heart get clogged, that's a recipe for a heart attack. If veins and arteries in your brain get blocked, that can cause a stroke. Clogged veins and arteries are a recipe for disaster.

There's also a pesky compound called TMAO (trimethylamine N-oxide) that we should talk about. Carnivores might not have heard about this, but it's a compound that our body produces when we digest certain nutrients found in meat. Studies have linked high levels of TMAO to a greater risk of heart attack and stroke. It's one of those things you don't want to be high in.

Moreover, it gets worse when you look at processed meats. Your beloved bacon, sausages, and deli slices are associated with even higher risks. The fat content, salt, and preservatives in them compound the problem, raising your blood pressure and doing a number on your arteries. The words 'heart health' and 'processed meat' really shouldn't be in the same sentence unless it's a warning.

Let's not forget inflammation. Chronic inflammation is like a smoldering fire in your body, and meat, particularly red and processed meat, is like kindling for that fire.

It can lead to atherosclerosis, where plaque builds up in your arteries, narrowing them and making a stroke or heart attack much more likely. It's a slow burn that can suddenly turn catastrophic.

In contrast to all these diseases from eating meat, plants have an amazing superpower where they actually help guard your heart. Unlike their meaty counterparts, plants are chock-full of fiber, antioxidants, and compounds that actively work to reduce inflammation and cholesterol levels. It's like they're patrolling the arteries, keeping them clear of the bad guys.

Our bodies were not designed for the meat-heavy diets that have become so common. In some parts of the world where they consume meat in only small quantities or use it as a side dish, those regions often see lower rates of heart disease and stroke. There's a lesson here: Perhaps more isn't always better.

But, 'What about protein?' In case you missed it in Chapter 3, protein is vital, but meat isn't the only source - not by a long shot. Plants provide protein, too, without all the risky baggage meat carries. Favoring plant-based protein sources can decrease your risk for those dreaded heart conditions.

Evidence is mounting, and it really can't be ignored any longer that a plant-based diet is the way to go for many reasons. Choosing plants over meat isn't just about personal preferences or ethical choices; it's a potent weapon in the fight against heart disease and stroke. These diseases can drastically alter the course of your life (or end it), and opting for plant power can be a life-saving decision. Seriously.

Going Green with your food choices is trendy and a strategic move for longevity and vitality. Heart disease and stroke don't have to be inevitable. Making the shift toward a plant-based diet could be the kindest thing you ever do for your heart and brain. And hey, the rest of your body - and the planet - will thank you, too.

Meat's Role in Diabetes Onset

When we consider what's on our plates, our taste buds and appetites generally dictate our choices. But let's dig deeper and see how these choices, particularly when they include a significant amount of meat, can affect our health.

Specifically, let's unravel the tangled threads connecting meat consumption to the onset of diabetes.

Type 2 diabetes is a complex chronic condition that has been spreading at an alarming rate. Lifestyle factors, including diet, play a huge role here. I know it's comfortable to cling to the familiar touchstones of traditional diets that often center around meat. Still, the connection between high meat intake and increased diabetes risk is too significant to ignore.

First, processed and red meat are loaded with saturated fats. The issue here is twofold - the fats can lead to weight gain and affect insulin sensitivity directly. As the body becomes less sensitive to insulin, it needs more to help glucose enter the cells. Eventually, the pancreas can't keep up, and blood sugar levels rise.

But it's not just the fat content we need to worry about; it's also the presence of advanced glycation end products or AGEs. These compounds are formed when meat is cooked at high temperatures, a standard preparation method. AGEs can cause inflammation and oxidative stress, which contribute to diabetes.

Processed meats, those that are smoked or cured, are particularly insidious. They contain nitrates and other preservatives tied to insulin resistance and even to the destruction of insulin-producing cells in the pancreas. While the research is still emerging, the correlation is too strong to dismiss.

Remember, meats (especially red and processed meats) often come with hefty amounts of sodium and other additives that can raise blood pressure and stress your blood vessels. Over time, this vascular onslaught can hamper the delivery of insulin and glucose to where they're needed, setting the stage for diabetes.

What about iron, specifically heme iron, which is abundant in red meat?

Our bodies need iron but in the right kind and amount. Too much heme iron can act as a pro-oxidant, damaging cells and tissues, including those involved in insulin production and regulation. Elevated body iron stores have been consistently linked with an increased risk of type 2 diabetes.

We've explored some ways that meat can be a one-way ticket to a less-than-desirable health destination, and the evidence is stacked. With meat-heavy diets driving up the risk of not just diabetes but a whole host of other health conditions, it can be easy to feel a bit overwhelmed.

But here's the silver lining: We've got the power to make choices that significantly reduce these risks. Transitioning to plant-based diets rich in whole foods like legumes, whole grains, fruits, and vegetables can guard against diabetes. Plants are packed with fiber, which helps control blood sugar, and their low glycemic index doesn't spike insulin levels.

Moreover, a plant-based diet is naturally lower in calories, helping maintain a healthy weight - a prominent factor in diabetes prevention. By pulling back from meat and embracing plants, we nurture our bodies with a wealth of micronutrients and phytochemicals that work harmoniously to keep our cells responsive and resilient to insulin.

In the grand tapestry of nutrition and health outcomes, it's essential to recognize the strings that tie our dietary patterns to conditions like diabetes.

Meat consumption has its place in dietary history, but the modern context (with its processed and heavy doses of animal products), has twisted it into a risk factor we can't afford to ignore.

For a path back to wellness, plants point the way forward, offering a blueprint for health that is as potent as it is palatable. Rethinking our plates today translates to a healthier, brighter tomorrow.

Other Health Risks and Diseases

When we think about meat consumption and its adverse effects, heart disease, strokes, and diabetes often jump to the forefront.

However, the rabbit hole of health concerns related to a meat-centered diet goes even deeper. In deciphering the vast array of additional risks, we perceive an intricate web of diseases that meat consumption may exacerbate or even initiate.

It's like navigating through a minefield, unaware of the hidden dangers lurking beneath the surface.

Let's talk about cancer and not just the types everyone is somewhat familiar with.

We've heard about the connections between red meat and colon cancer. But there are more layers to this. For instance, consuming processed meats has been linked to an increased risk of stomach and pancreatic cancer.

Certain compounds in meat (especially when preserved or cooked at high temperatures) can form carcinogens.

What about switching to white meats like chicken or fish? Unfortunately, they are not entirely off the hook either; emerging evidence suggests they may also be implicated in various health issues when consumed in excess.

Now, let's move from the gut to the kidneys: Our bean-shaped friends do an incredible job filtering and cleaning our blood, but they can be overwhelmed by the onslaught of animal proteins.

High meat consumption can lead to an increased risk of kidney stones and even chronic kidney disease over time. If we think of proteins as bricks for the body's construction, it's like dumping in more bricks than the workers (in this case, our kidneys) can handle, eventually leading to a disastrous pile-up.

Rheumatoid arthritis is another concern, sneaking up on individuals through stiff and inflamed joints. While it's a complex autoimmune condition, studies hint that a meat-heavy diet might increase susceptibility or worsen symptoms. This doesn't mean cutting out meat will cure arthritis overnight, but it might make the difference between a manageable condition and one that significantly disrupts your life.

Then, we have the impact on our respiratory system - a lesser-known concern: Asthma, for instance, can be aggravated by a high-meat diet due to increased inflammation levels in the body. Imagine the foods you consume clouding your lungs like smog muddies a clear sky. Not a pleasant thought, right?

And don't get me started on the links between meat and conditions like sleep apnea. It's a bit like trying to sleep with a band blasting in the next room - the excess weight from a high-meat diet potentially contributes to fatty deposits around the neck area, which can obstruct your airways.

Now, if you consider yourself a brainiac or value your cognitive function, heed this: studies are now highlighting the connection between meat-heavy diets and risks for neurodegenerative diseases like Alzheimer's.

That's right; what you eat can influence your brain's destiny. It's as if meat is a Trojan horse for these ailments, sneaking up on your precious neurons under the guise of a hearty meal.

Let's now glance at the invisible enemy named 'antibiotic resistance.' The rampant overuse of antibiotics in livestock to promote growth and prevent disease in often overcrowded conditions has a spillover effect. It's giving rise to superbugs that are tougher to treat, which means the steak on your plate might be a silent contributor to a global health crisis.

Finally, there are infertility concerns and hormonal disruptions, particularly pressing for future parents out there. Hormones and other additives in meat can interfere with your body's natural balance, throwing a wrench into reproductive plans. It's as if each bite of hormone-laden meat is tossing a pebble on the delicate scales of your endocrine system.

The solution to avoiding this cocktail of health hazards is transitioning toward a more plant-based diet that can be an elixir, offering a cornucopia of health benefits while sidestepping the dark alleyways meat can lead us down.

Remember, while our dietary choices have profound personal implications, there's a spectrum of bodily systems quietly depending on those decisions. We can support them best by opting for the world of greens, grains, legumes, and fruits - the natural palate of preventative medicine.

In essence, pivoting away from meat and towards plants isn't simply about dodging heart disease or diabetes. It's about respecting the complexity of our body's systems and giving them the best chance to thrive. As we'll explore in upcoming chapters, a whole-food, plant-based diet isn't just a preventative measure; it's a proactive step towards a vibrant, disease-resistant life.

So, let's leave behind the silent saboteurs lurking in meat and embrace the power of plants, the true champions of our health.

Chapter 5: The Plant-Based Advantage

Let's dive in and explore the remarkable benefits of a diet grounded in greens and whole grains.

It's not just about what we're missing by avoiding meat; it's about what we're gaining from the earth's cornucopia of plants. A plant-based diet teems with a kaleidoscope of vitamins and minerals, often playing second fiddle in conversations dominated by protein.

But here's the big reveal: plant foods are incredibly nutrient-dense, meaning they pack a ton of nutrition in relatively few calories. This isn't just good news; it's great news for anyone looking to nourish their body without overloading it.

Think of every bite as a step towards revitalizing your health, where leafy greens, vibrant vegetables, hearty legumes, and succulent fruits take center stage in your dietary lineup.

Beyond basic nutrients, plants are our premium source for an array of phytochemicals and antioxidants - those unsung heroes in the nutrition narrative. They're the compounds that plants use to protect themselves, and when we eat these plants, their armor becomes our armor.

As antioxidants combat free radicals, reducing oxidative stress, phytochemicals quietly work to bolster our immune system, tune up our cardiovascular function, and even influence the mechanisms underlying chronic diseases. It's like having a personal health entourage, courtesy of every plant-based meal. And remember, these benefits aren't just theoretical - they're tangible, studied, and well-documented boosts to our well-being.

Pay attention to the fiber factor, too. It's a game-changer for health and a powerhouse for prevention. Plant-based eaters experience the magic of fiber with each meal - it regulates digestion, supports a healthy gut microbiome (and keeps things moving) if you know what I mean. But the true beauty of fiber lies in its fullness factor and its role in disease prevention.

Unlike meat, plants provide this essential nutrient, which has been linked to lower rates of heart disease, type 2 diabetes, and even certain cancers.

So, there you have it: the plant-based advantage is like hitting the jackpot for your body, bringing together a wealth of nutrients, defending champions against oxidation, and the fantastic fiber that keeps us feeling great. Now, isn't that a meal deal you just can't beat?

Nutrient Density and Diversity

Embarking on a journey through plant-based eating brings us to an essential aspect of nutrition: the powerful duo of nutrient density and diversity.

Imagine filling your plate with a kaleidoscope of fruits, veggies, legumes, seeds, and whole grains. Not only are you creating an art piece, but you're also crafting a health fortress with each meal. But what is this talk of nutrient density, and why should your taste buds and body care so much?

Nutrient density refers to the amount of beneficial nutrients packed into a given volume or weight of food. Think of it like an enriching bang for your dietary buck. Plant-based foods excel in this, offering vitamins, minerals, and other health-promoting substances in spades without the unnecessary baggage of excess calories or harmful fats. This way, you can eat more, feel satiated yet light, and fuel your body optimally.

Diversity is the sidekick to density, creating a spectrum of nutrients that work synergistically within your body. It's not just about eating your greens but also your reds, purples, oranges, and yellows.

Each color often represents different nutrients and phytochemicals right at home in a plant eater's palette. So when you reach for that vibrant array, you're not just making your plate more inviting; you're ensuring that your body receives a comprehensive suite of health-promoting compounds.

The diversity found in plants goes beyond the visible. Fiber, for example, isn't just a single entity. There are various types (soluble, insoluble, fermentable) that play distinct roles within your body, from regulating blood sugar to promoting a healthy gut flora.

And let's remember the myriad of plant proteins are not only sufficient but often superior due to their accompanying nutrients and lack of adverse health associations found in meat.

Eating a diet rich in plant foods ensures that you're meeting both macro and micro requirements. These micro-nutrients are often unsung heroes, supporting enzyme function, protecting against oxidative stress, and bolstering your immune system.

With plants, you're addressing your hunger and caring for your holistic health, one cell at a time.

The concern often arises: can I get enough of everything my body needs from plants alone? The answer is a resounding yes. With planning and a bit of knowledge, a varied plant-based diet can cover all your nutritional bases. This might mean munching on Brazil nuts for selenium, red bell peppers for vitamin C, or chia seeds for omega-3s, but that's hardly a chore when each bite is ripe with flavor and goodness.

Some people worry about the absence of meat equating to a lack of diversity or that eating only plants is somehow inferior or unhealthy. However, the opposite is true.

The plant kingdom boasts tens of thousands of edible wonders, many of which pack a nutritional punch unrivaled by a slab of steak. When you swap out meat for plant-based options, you're not losing out; you're unlocking a treasure chest of diverse nutrients the Earth has to offer.

A plant-based diet offers the freedom to explore and enjoy a wide variety of foods. By consistently mixing things up, you not only prevent dietary boredom but also cover more nutritional ground. Think lentils one night, quinoa the next, followed by wild rice; it's an adventure for your taste buds and a godsend for your well-being.

Moreover, embracing nutrient density and diversity can have a profound effect on combating chronic diseases. Many plants contain bioactive compounds that may reduce inflammation, improve lipid profiles, and stabilize blood glucose levels. This adds a layer of disease prevention that might be compromised when meals are heavy on meat and light on plants.

As our exploration of the plant-based advantage continues, the importance of nutrient density and diversity becomes apparent. It's about getting the most nutritional bang for your buck while reveling in a variety of tastes and textures.

It's a testament to how a diet abundant in plant-based foods can be both a joy to eat and a cornerstone for optimal health. So, let's cherish the variety and dig into the nutritional powerhouse that plant-based living is – your body and taste buds will thank you for it.

Phytochemicals and Antioxidants

As we journey deeper into the plant-based adventure, let's take a moment to spotlight some of the unsung nutrition heroes: phytochemicals and antioxidants.

These compounds give plants their vibrant colors and distinctive flavors, and they also wield the power to protect our health in profound ways. Here's the breakdown of why they're integral to a plant-based diet and how they stand in stark contrast to meat-centered eating habits.

Phytochemicals are natural compounds found in plants that, while not essential for our survival, have significant health benefits. They're like plant superpowers, with each type offering unique advantages. You've likely heard of some, like flavonoids in blueberries, lycopene in tomatoes, and resveratrol in red grapes. These biologically active molecules help defend against chronic diseases and support our well-being in many ways.

Antioxidants are the bodyguards against oxidative stress, a process that can lead to cell damage and plays a part in various diseases. They're like little scavengers, hunting down free radicals (the troublemakers of our bodies) and neutralizing them. Fortunately, plant foods are packed with these protective antioxidants, from vitamins C and E to minerals like selenium.

This is important when considering a plant-based diet over its meaty counterpart because meat simply can't offer the same array of phytochemicals and antioxidants.

Plant foods provide a complex cocktail of these compounds, working synergistically to enhance their individual effects. It's like having an entire team of superheroes on your side, compared to the lone-ranger approach of a meat-heavy diet.

Take, for example, the carotenoids - a group of phytochemicals that include beta-carotene, lutein, and zeaxanthin. These not only give carrots and sweet potatoes their orange hue, but they're also stellar for eye health.

And then there's the army of antioxidants found in dark leafy greens, nuts, and seeds that work to reduce inflammation, which is at the heart of many chronic health issues.

Studies have linked high antioxidant intake to a reduced risk of heart disease and certain cancers. It's imperative to understand that while the body can fend off free radicals to an extent, the additional support from a diet rich in antioxidants can be a game-changer for long-term health.

If you're thinking about the volume and variety of phytochemicals necessary, rest easy knowing that a diverse plant-based diet naturally encompasses a broad spectrum of these powerful substances. Every meal is an opportunity to fuel your body with a different phytochemical profile.

All the angles are covered, from the L-arginine in nuts that helps your blood vessels relax to the anthocyanins in berries that support brain health.

Another point worth noting is the environment within our gut. Phytochemicals and antioxidants from plants nourish the vast community of beneficial microbes. Good gut health is linked to enhanced immunity, improved mood, and reduced risk of various diseases, something a meat-centered diet (lacking these components) often neglects.

It's all about embracing the naturally occurring pharmacy in our plant friends. By loading up on fruits, vegetables, legumes, whole grains, and nuts, we're not just meeting our nutrient quotas but exceeding them. It's like equipping the body with an arsenal of health-promoting compounds that protect against the onslaught of modern-era diseases, and that's something meat can't compete with.

In closing, ingesting a vast array of phytochemicals and antioxidants is not just about prevention; it's a proactive approach to enhance our life force. A plant-based diet shines a spotlight on these compounds, enabling us to thrive, not just survive.

Consuming plants is a direct pipeline to this treasure trove of wellness, so let's harness the power of plants to energize, protect, and revitalize our bodies in each delicious bite.

Now that we've highlighted the crucial roles of phytochemicals and antioxidants let's prepare to delve into another cornerstone of plant-based well-being - the fiber factor and its potent impact on health. Stay tuned as we uncover more about how the elements of a plant-based diet contribute to an optimal health picture.

The Fiber Factor in Health

As we delve into the myriad of benefits offered by a plant-based diet, let's not overlook the superhero of nutrition: Fiber. Humble and often underrated, dietary fiber is a power player in maintaining and improving health.

While protein often hogs the nutritional spotlight, fiber offers a cascade of health perks.

But here's a twist - Fiber is only found in plant foods. This critical component is glaringly absent from meat and other animal products, which is something to chew on for those still sitting on the fence about plant-based nutrition.

Fiber works its magic through a few mechanisms. First, it plays a role in digestion and weight management. High-fiber foods are more filling, keeping you satisfied longer and reducing the urge for seconds or thirds. They also tend to be lower in calories than their nutrient density - a win-win for those looking to maintain or lose weight without the gnawing pangs of hunger.

However, the benefits of fiber extend well beyond feeling full. Fiber acts like a broom for your digestive tract, sweeping through and helping flush out waste and toxins. This process helps to keep you regular and reduces the risk of developing diverticular disease. Think of it as internal housekeeping that keeps things running smoothly and the pipes clean day in and day out.

Additionally, a fiber-rich diet has been consistently linked to lower cholesterol levels.

Soluble Fiber, found in oats, nuts, seeds, and many fruits and vegetables, binds to cholesterol particles in your digestive system and helps to remove them from your body. This natural cholesterol management is particularly compelling regarding heart health, placing fiber in the limelight for those paying attention to their cardiovascular well-being.

Moreover, fiber is your gut bacteria's favorite meal. As it ferments in the gut, it produces short-chain fatty acids with potent anti-inflammatory properties. This action is not just beneficial for digestive health; mounting evidence suggests it plays a role in reducing the risk of chronic diseases such as type 2 diabetes and certain cancers. In short, a fiber-rich diet is one of the best things you can do for your gut microbiome (your body's internal ecosystem).

Managing blood sugar is another lesser-sung verse in fiber's praise song. Those who prefer plant-based eating will find that the fiber in whole grains, legumes, and vegetables helps slow the absorption of sugar, leading to a more gradual rise in blood sugar levels. It's a natural approach to maintaining energy levels and preventing those infamous sugar highs and crashes, which no one is fond of.

But let's not forget the protective bubble fiber forms against various forms of cancer. Studies have shown a clear association between high dietary fiber intake and a reduced risk of colorectal cancer. It turns out that fiber's role in moving waste through your digestive system does more than contribute to overall comfort; it helps protect against disease.

In the age of a supplement-obsessed culture, it's important to remember that fiber is best obtained through whole plant foods, not just a powder or a pill.

The absorption of vitamins and minerals from supplements is very low; our bodies have a much easier time getting vitamins from their sources in a whole-food package.

Additionally, vitamins work in concert with other source factors instead of being extracted and isolated. In other words, it is much better for your body to eat an entire apple or orange than trying to take a vitamin C supplement.

Fiber is an essential component of plant foods and brings other beneficial nutrients like vitamins, minerals, and antioxidants. This synergistic effect of whole foods is something that isolated supplements cannot mimic.

With these benefits in mind, it's easy to see why a plant-based diet promotes health.

Whether you're talking about longevity, disease prevention, or everyday vitality, the fiber factor plays a crucial role. It's no flash in the pan - Fiber is the steady drumbeat of a plant-based diet, laying down a rhythm for a life of wellness.

So, as you think about your next meal, consider how you can up the ante on your fiber intake. A bowl of lentil soup, a hearty salad, an apple, or some raspberries are not just a meal's components but are investments in your long-term health.

Embrace the plant-based advantage, and let fiber-packed foods pave your path to lasting vitality.

Chapter 6: Fat Facts - Omega Balance and Cholesterol

We're venturing into some seriously misunderstood territory when we talk about fats.

The kind of fats we consume, especially when it comes to omega fatty acids, play a crucial role in our overall heart health. Hold on; before you think I'm going to rave about omega-3s and bash all the rest, it's essential to grasp the concept of balance.

Our bodies are incredible machines that need a mix of omega-3 and omega-6 fatty acids but in the right proportion. It's all about that delicate see-saw of nutritional equilibrium. And guess what? A plant-based diet sets you up for this balance beautifully, providing a symphony of sources like flaxseeds, chia seeds, and walnuts without overdoing it.

But let's not stop there. The buzzword cholesterol often pops up with a red alarm attached to it. However, you'll find that staying within a greener pasture can keep these levels in check, thanks to minimal saturated fats and no dietary cholesterol found in plants.

You see, while your body needs a little bit of cholesterol for proper function (and can make it), it's the type and amount that matters. However, eating animals is a VIP pass for saturated fats to wreak havoc, doing the cholesterol two-step right into your arteries.

In contrast, embracing a plant-based diet is like choosing the slow, rhythmic dance of health - highlighting unsaturated fats, which have the neat trick of actually helping to lower bad cholesterol levels.

Plus, plants come with a bonus: fiber! It's not just the ruffage keeping things smooth in the digestive dance floor; it's also grabbing onto excess cholesterol and inviting it right out the door. By choosing plants, you're winning the cholesterol game with every bite.

Plant-Based Sources of Essential Fatty Acids

Let's dive right into one of the most vibrant corners of plant-based nutrition: essential fatty acids (EFAs).

Omegas - you've probably heard that word tossed around regarding fats. Specifically, we're talking about Omega-3 and Omega-6 fatty acids. These guys are like the VIPs of the fatty world; your body can't make them, so you've got to include them in your diet.

People often think of fish when they hear Omega-3s, but let's shine a light on the plant kingdom where these nutrients thrive without the fishy middleman.

First up, **flaxseeds**. These little seeds are powerhouses, rich in alpha-linolenic acid (ALA), an Omega-3 fatty acid. When you sprinkle flaxseed onto your cereal or whirl it into your smoothies, you're not just adding a nutty flavor but delivering a nutrient boost that your body will convert into the Omega-3 fats it needs. And while you're at it, remember **chia seeds** and **hemp seeds**, which are equally fantastic sources of ALA and pack a punch for fiber and protein, too.

Walnuts are another fantastic plant-based source. They're a snack that's as heart-friendly as they are tasty. A handful a day gives you a significant amount of ALA and contributes to a well-rounded, cholesterol-friendly diet. For those who might be nuts about nuts, walnuts are an easy addition to your daily menu.

Let's talk **leafy greens**. Spinach, kale, and Brussels sprouts may not be the titans of EFAs that seeds and nuts are, but they still contribute to your Omega-3 intake. It's all about the greens. These veggies serve as a reminder that good things come in all packages – even the leafy, green ones. Every bite is a step toward a balanced Omega profile.

Now, onto a culinary favorite: the **avocado**. Creamy, delicious, and chock-full of Omega-3s and monounsaturated fats – the kind that cheers your heart on. Avocado is versatile, making it an easy addition to any meal. It's like nature's butter but with a resume that outshines any dairy product.

Transitioning a bit here, let's consider the power of **soy**. Edamame, tofu, and tempeh aren't just substitutions for meat; they're a source of Omega-6 and Omega-3, providing a balance that helps guide your body toward better health. Plus, they're delectable in a myriad of dishes!

For the oil connoisseurs, let's talk about some plant-based oils that are fabulous for your fatty acid balance. **Canola oil**, for instance, boasts a friendly ratio of Omega-6 to Omega-3, giving it a thumbs-up for heart health. Similarly, **flaxseed oil** holds its weight in ALA content, so it's another grand option for dressings or drizzling over your favorite meals.

We can't forget about **algae**. Maybe it doesn't make your mouth water like ripe avocado, but algae oil is a gold mine for DHA and EPA – types of Omega-3s found in fish.

Guess what? *Fish get them from eating algae, so why not skip the fish and go straight to the source?* Algae-based supplements are also a sustainable choice for those conscious about ocean life and ecosystems.

Here's the key takeaway: implementing a cornucopia of these plant-based options into your diet can easily fulfill your body's essential fatty acid needs. It's not just about dodging the meat; it's about embracing an abundance of flavors and nutrients in whole, plant-based foods. Your body will thank you with better Omega balance, and so will your taste buds.

To wrap it up, Omega balance is critical for maintaining heart health and overall wellness.

And while meat has historically been a go-to source for EFAs, it isn't the only way, or dare I say, not even the best way.

The plant kingdom is brimming with sources that can support our health without the risks associated with high cholesterol and saturated fat in meats. By welcoming plant-based sources of EFAs into your diet, you're opening the door to improved health and an appreciation for the rich variety plants offer.

The Impact of Saturated Fat from Meat

Now, let's talk about a hot topic often sizzling on the grill of nutritional debates: saturated fat from meat.

Sure, a juicy steak might seem irresistible for many folks, but when it comes to health, it's loaded with saturated fats, which, let's face it, have a less-than-stellar reputation. The truth is that the saturated fat found in meat can be a real troublemaker for our bodies, especially for our heart health.

The Good, The Bad, The Ugly (Cholesterol)

For starters, saturated fat raises low-density lipoprotein (LDL) cholesterol, the type of cholesterol you've probably heard called 'bad.'

This is because LDL cholesterol can build up on the walls of your arteries, forming plaque that makes them narrow and less flexible - a condition known as atherosclerosis. This can set the stage for heart attacks and strokes, turning that fleeting pleasure of a fatty meal into a long-term health gamble.

In other words, cholesterol is necessary for various physiological processes, but excessive cholesterol levels in the blood can increase the risk of cardiovascular diseases such as heart disease and stroke.

For simplicity, think of it like this: There are two kinds of cholesterol - good (HDL) and bad (LDL). But first, let me explain what cholesterol is exactly.

All mammals, including humans, produce cholesterol (the good kind, HDL). Cholesterol is a vital lipid molecule that plays crucial roles in cell membrane structure, hormone synthesis, and bile acid production. It is synthesized primarily in the liver but also in other tissues throughout the body. Cholesterol is essential for the proper functioning of cells and is transported in the bloodstream in lipoprotein particles.

So that's 'the good cholesterol' our bodies make, need, and use naturally. The 'bad cholesterol' is the excess cholesterol we get from consuming other animals.

Our bodies are miraculous at metabolizing cholesterol in moderation, but true carnivores are even better at it. In fact, lions, tigers, cheetahs, etc., do not get heart attacks and strokes to the degree that humans do because they can process the bad cholesterol much better than humans. That alone should be enough to convince you that we are not carnivores, but let me give you the scientific explanation real quick:

Carnivores, primarily consuming animal-based foods (meat), are naturally exposed to dietary cholesterol from their prey. They have efficient mechanisms to regulate cholesterol synthesis and metabolism to accommodate their higher dietary cholesterol intake. Their bodies can adjust cholesterol production and absorption to maintain a balance suited to their nutritional needs.

In contrast, herbivores have digestive systems and metabolic processes optimized for processing plant-based foods and managing lower cholesterol levels compared to carnivores.

Instead, they obtain essential lipids from plant sources and have different strategies to meet their nutritional requirements. Therefore, if an herbivore consumes animal-based foods or ingests excessive amounts of cholesterol, it is not a natural part of an herbivore's diet and can potentially lead to health issues.

While a single instance of consuming animal-based foods may not necessarily be immediately harmful to an herbivore, regular consumption of such foods or exposure to high levels of dietary cholesterol could disrupt their digestive processes and metabolic balance over time. Depending on the species and specific circumstances, This could lead to digestive upset, nutrient imbalances, and other health complications.

In extreme cases, consuming large amounts of animal-based foods or excessive cholesterol could potentially lead to acute health problems **or even death in herbivores**.

However, it's important to note that such scenarios would be highly unusual in natural environments where herbivores have access to their typical plant-based diets and are not exposed to high levels of dietary cholesterol.

Overall, while herbivores are not adapted to consuming animal-based foods or processing high levels of cholesterol, the occasional accidental ingestion of small amounts is unlikely to be immediately life-threatening. However, long-term exposure to such foods or high cholesterol levels could impact their health and well-being.

Fatty Acids

Let's remember the balance of our omegas, too. Our bodies are crying out for omega-3 and omega-6 fatty acids in a harmonious balance, and meat throws a wrench in this plan.

Meat is typically high in omega-6 and low in omega-3, which can tilt the scales toward inflammation in our bodies, setting off a domino effect of health issues.

Furthermore, meat isn't just about fats; it's also about what's missing. When you opt for meat, especially in large quantities, you might be missing out on other essential nutrients that plant-based sources of fat, such as avocados or nuts, bring to the table in abundance. These plants offer healthier fats and a suite of vitamins, minerals, and fibers critical for maintaining optimal health.

Omega-3 and omega-6 are polyunsaturated fatty acids (PUFAs), essential fats that the body needs for various physiological functions. These fatty acids are essential because the body cannot produce them independently and must obtain them from the diet.

Omega-3 fatty acids are a group of fatty acids known for their anti-inflammatory properties and numerous health benefits.

The three main types of omega-3 fatty acids are:

- Alpha-linolenic acid (ALA): Found primarily in plant-based sources such as flaxseeds, chia seeds, walnuts, and leafy green vegetables.

- Eicosapentaenoic acid (EPA): Found primarily in fatty fish such as salmon, mackerel, and sardines, *as well as certain algae supplements.*

- Docosahexaenoic acid (DHA): Also found primarily in fatty fish *and certain algae supplements*, DHA is particularly important for brain function and eye health.

Omega-6 fatty acids are another group of essential fatty acids that play important roles in the body's inflammatory response and various physiological processes. The main type of omega-6 fatty acid is linoleic acid (LA), which is abundant in vegetable oils such as soybean, corn, and sunflower.

Both omega-3 and omega-6 fatty acids are important for overall health, but the balance between these two types of fatty acids is crucial.

In the typical Western diet, omega-6 to omega-3 fatty acids are often skewed toward omega-6 fatty acids (because it is mainly acquired from eating animals), which can contribute to chronic inflammation and various health problems.

Therefore, it's essential to regularly consume sources of omega-3 fatty acids and maintain a balanced intake of omega-3 and omega-6 fatty acids for optimal health.

In Closing

What's concerning, too, is that the conversation about meat and saturated fats often eclipses an equally significant issue: **processed meats**. They're not just high in fats; they're a carnival of added sodium, preservatives, and sometimes sugars, which pile on additional health risks.

But it's not all doom and gloom. The beauty is you can take control. By reducing or eliminating meat intake (and instead indulging in rich plant-based sources of healthier fats), you can help maintain more favorable cholesterol levels and support a healthy inflammatory response.

Think of it as a well-oiled machine versus one running with a sputter - obviously, you'd prefer the former.

Some might argue, 'But meat's been on our plates for centuries!' Sure, but back then, the animals weren't jam-packed with the chemicals and hormones that today's industrial farming practices use.

Plus, our ancestors didn't have meat as frequently or in the proportions we do today.

Moderation and the quality of meat consumed back then were quite different from what we see in most modern diets.

To paint a clearer picture, regularly consuming high amounts of regular and processed meat has been associated with an array of chronic diseases, including certain types of cancer.

Not to rain on the parade, but it's important to recognize that what's on your fork can significantly affect your long-term wellness.

Transitioning to a more plant-dominated diet paves the way for improved health. You're eliminating the risks associated with saturated fat from meat and infusing your body with a spectrum of protective nutrients found in plants. And in the long run, this shift can help maintain a healthier body weight and a more robust immune system.

So, yes, while that steak might be calling your name, remember that there's a symphony of flavors and health benefits waiting for you in the plant kingdom. It's a choice that your taste buds and your body will thank you for as you journey toward a heart-healthy and vibrant lifestyle.

Chapter 7: Plant-Powered Endurance and Athleticism

When we dive into the world of sports and fitness, there's an ever-growing community of athletes swearing by the benefits of a plant-based diet.

They're not just embracing greens and grains for the planet's sake but for a competitive edge. It may not be the consensus yet, but the examples are compelling enough to turn our attention to the potential of plant-powered performance.

Let's face it; there's a reason why some of the fittest and most resilient athletes are choosing kale over kebabs. It goes beyond ethical choices and connects deeply with how our bodies handle and thrive on various fuel types.

The secret to superior endurance might be nestled in that humble bowl of lentils or that vibrant, antioxidant-rich berry smoothie.

What if I told you that swapping steak for spinach could do wonders for your stamina?

Skeptical?

Given the meat-centered paradigm of athleticism we've been fed for decades, it's understandable.

However, evidence suggests that loading up on plants can enhance blood flow, reduce inflammation, and speed up recovery. What you eat can nudge you from merely finishing the race to scaling the upper echelons of athletic prowess.

And let's pay attention to the hydration and micronutrients packed in fruits and veggies, which can support sustained energy levels during grueling workouts or competitions.

Whether for your heartbeats per minute or the sheer love of pushing your limits, nourishing your system with various plants could be the winning ticket. It's not just about protein; it's about a symphony of nutrients working in concert to keep your engine running smoothly.

Imagine tackling your fitness goals with a diet that's kind to your body and the planet. It's not a whimsical dream but a tangible, reachable state when powered by plants.

So maybe the next time you're pondering how to improve your game, consider this: The plant kingdom might be the most underrated team member in your athletic arsenal.

Historical Examples of Plant-Fueled Athletes

When we delve into the annals of athletic history, we find a rich tapestry of individuals who have thrived and excelled on plant-centered diets. These pioneers of plant-powered athleticism provide compelling evidence that optimal performance isn't exclusive to those who consume carnivorous fare.

Take, for instance, the ancient gladiators of Rome, often called the "Barley Men." You might think they'd feast on meat to maintain their fierce reputation in the arena, but historical records suggest these athletes primarily consumed grains and legumes. Their plant-based diet was substantial enough to sustain rigorous training and brutal combat, debunking the notion that meat is the only path to peak physical condition.

Moving centuries forward, the Tarahumara people of Mexico's Copper Canyons have long been renowned for their extraordinary long-distance running abilities. They exist on a traditional diet deeply rooted in maize, beans, and other plant staples. Rich in complex carbohydrates and low in fat, this diet powers their incredible endurance, proving a meat-heavy menu isn't mandatory for extraordinary athletic prowess.

The legendary Paavo Nurmi, a Finnish middle-distance and long-distance runner, dominated his competitions from 1920 to the 1930s. Known as the "Flying Finn," Nurmi credited his success partly to a diet devoid of meat, emphasizing how plants can fuel sustained athletic success. As his career progressed, he leaned more into his vegetarian diet, finding benefits in his performance and recovery.

Turning to sports of brawn, six-time Mr. Olympia winner Bill Pearl switched to a vegetarian diet midway through his bodybuilding career during the 1950s-1960s. His continued successes laid the foundation for a growing wave of plant-based bodybuilders and strength athletes who challenge the stereotype that meat is essential for building substantial muscle mass. Mr. Pearl passed away in 2022 at the age of 91 years old.

A name that reverberates in the walls of martial arts history is that of Edwin J. Brady, known as "The Vegetarian Boxer." In the early 1900s, Brady maintained an undefeated streak while following a strict vegetarian diet, casting aside doubts about plant-based nutrition's ability to nourish the explosive agility and strength required in the boxing ring.

What about endurance? The remarkable Fiona Oakes, an elite marathon runner, set multiple records and even won the North Pole Marathon. Her feats are all the more impressive when considering her strict vegan diet since she was six years old, which she's maintained alongside her athletic endeavors, sending a powerful message about endurance on plants.

In competitive cycling, where stamina and energy are kings, the Belgian rider Eddy Merckx, known as "The Cannibal" for his voracious appetite for victory (and not for meat), frequently opted for a predominantly plant-based diet, particularly before his races. His triumphant career, boasting an astonishing 525 victories, highlights how plant nutrition adequately supports even the most demanding endurance sports.

Then there's Dave Scott, one of the most recognized triathletes, known for winning the Ironman World Championship six times. A vegetarian diet fueled his performance during his peak competing years in the 1980s-1990s. Scott's achievement suggests that even in the grueling triathlon conditions, plant-based nutrition doesn't just suffice; it excels.

Lastly, let's talk about the powerhouse of Charlene Wong Williams – a Canadian figure skater who competed in the Winter Olympics. She graced the ice with elegance and endurance while maintaining a vegetarian diet since the age of fifteen. Her success on national and international stages underlines the power of plants in even the most artistic and demanding sports, where energy and mental clarity are inseparable.

While the tales of these individuals run far and wide across various disciplines, they all converge on a singular truth: a plant-based diet is a viable, often advantageous, fuel for athletes. These historical figures were not just exceptions to the rule; they were trailblazers who illustrated the boundless potential of plants in nurturing physical excellence.

Their legacies testify to the profound impact of choosing greens over grains, legumes over sirloins, and fruits over fillets - turning plant power into a timeless ally for athletic triumph.

Modern-Day Plant-Based Performance

The conversation around athletes and nutrition is buzzing with the compelling case for a plant-based diet.

We are witnessing a veritable revolution where athletes at the pinnacle of their sports are surviving and thriving on diets free of animal products.

Gone are the days when the stereotype of a 'weak vegetarian' had any credence; today's plant-eaters are flipping the script. Plant-powered athletes are breaking records and taking names across various disciplines, from endurance sports like ultra-marathons to explosive power sports like weightlifting and professional football.

Consider the stamina of marathoners or triathletes who have swapped steak for spinach and are setting personal bests. These athletes have discovered that a meal rich in leafy greens, complex carbohydrates, and plant proteins leads to sustainable, long-term energy reserves. This bounty of nutrition supports extended periods of exertion, reduces recovery time, and slashes inflammation, steering clear of the chronic soreness that's all too familiar for many in the meat-eating cadre.

Let's take this discussion into the gym, where strength athletes pushing for peak performance are reaching for beans, nuts, and seeds as their source of protein. These muscle-building mavens (someone who is dazzlingly skilled) have debunked the antiquated notion that meat is essential for peak physical development. By fueling their bodies with plants, they achieve gains without the unwanted baggage of cholesterol and saturated fats that come with animal proteins.

Studies reinforce what these athletes are already demonstrating anecdotally: a plant-based diet can support and even enhance athletic performance. This diet increases blood flow and oxygen to the muscles, essentially upping the ante regarding endurance and power.

Furthermore, the antioxidants and phytonutrients prevalent in plant foods fight oxidative stress, meaning our plant-eating athletes are performing better today and paving the way for continued excellence well into the future.

But it's not just the physical benefits that are turning heads. Cognitive advantages like sharper focus and quicker reaction times are becoming a new frontier for plant-based diets in sports. The same nutrients that keep blood vessels clear and flowing in the body do the same for the brain, keeping it well-fueled and ready to make snap decisions that are crucial in competitive settings.

A discussion on modern-day plant-based performance wouldn't be complete without addressing the elephant in the room: the environment. Athletes are increasingly concerned with the sustainability and ethical implications of their diet. The lower environmental impact of a plant-based diet sits well with the ethos of many athletes who focus on personal health, performance, and a sustainable world.

From anecdotal evidence to scientific studies and environmental considerations, the reasons for switching to a plant-based lifestyle are stacking up.

It's a powerful indication that what we feed our bodies can either be a foundation for excellence or a barrier to it. For those seeking not only to excel in their athletic endeavors but also to lead a life that's in harmony with the world around them, the choice is getting more apparent with every stride on the track and each lift in the gym.

While these changes don't happen overnight, the trend is evident. Elite athletes vouch for the benefits of going green - not just in the literal sense with their food, but also figuratively with the medals and records to show for it. Many find that once they tune into their body's needs and answer with a kaleidoscope of plants, the body responds with a resounding yes, proving powerful and capable beyond what they once thought possible.

In the following chapters, we will delve deeper into the specifics of how this plant-based performance works. We'll explore the attributes of various macro and micronutrients that give plant-based diets their zest and examine how they empower athletes to manage weight, metabolism, and cognitive functions.

But for now, let's take inspiration from these modern-day gladiators of the sports world who show us that eating plants can provide the fuel needed for extraordinary performance.

Chapter 8: Weight Management and Metabolism

Lean into this: embracing a plant-based diet could be the game-changer you've been looking for in your weight management journey.

Sure, calories matter, but not all calories are created equal. The caloric density of plant foods is a hot topic, and for good reason. Packed with nutrients yet lower in calories, plant-based foods fill you up without weighing you down.

Imagine chowing down on a big bowl of veggie stew or a colorful salad. Your stomach feels full, and your body fueled, but you haven't blown your calorie budget for the day. This harmonious balance between intake and satisfaction is why plants are exceptionally proficient at helping individuals achieve and maintain a healthy weight.

But it's not just about the calories - it's also what's happening behind the scenes in your body. Plants come with a built-in fat loss ally: their impact on metabolism. Unlike heavily processed foods and fatty meat products that can stall your metabolism, whole plant foods keep that metabolic fire stoked.

High in fiber and complex carbohydrates, they take longer to digest, meaning your body must work harder and burn more energy to process them. This subtle yet steady revving of the metabolic engines aids in melting away unwanted fat and maintaining lean muscle mass, especially when combined with regular physical activity. It's like having a personal assistant for your metabolism, one rooting for your success around the clock.

Now, it's one thing to hear about the positive impacts of a plant-based diet on weight management, but living it is where the magic happens. By transitioning to meals rich in vegetables, fruits, legumes, whole grains, nuts, and seeds, you join a movement that's not just trimming waistlines but also reinforcing health from head to toe.

As you'll see, weight management is just one piece of the vibrant tapestry of benefits afforded by a plant-based diet, and understanding this comprehensive impact on metabolism can be a life-changing revelation.

As you focus on incorporating these vital foods, you're contributing to a leaner profile and paving the way for a vigorous, zestful life. With each plant-packed meal, you're taking control of your health destiny, one delicious bite at a time.

Caloric Density of Plant Foods

Caloric density is a game changer when it comes to losing weight or maintaining a healthy one. Imagine this: you can eat larger volumes of food, feel full, and consume fewer calories.

Sounds pretty ideal, right? Well, that's exactly what a plant-based diet offers. Most plant foods have a lower caloric density than animal products, which means you can enjoy your meals without worrying about overdoing them on calories.

Let me give you the breakdown of why this caloric density thing is a big deal. Picture a plate piled high with vibrant veggies, fruits bursting with color, hearty grains, and legumes. This plate isn't just a feast for the eyes; it's packed with nutrients but not overloaded with calories. These foods have fewer calories for their volume, so you can eat more and weigh less. That's like hitting the food jackpot!

How exactly does this work? Well, it's mostly down to water and fiber. Plant foods are typically high in both, which adds bulk without adding calories. This means you get that satisfying feeling of a full stomach, but you're not taking in a huge number of calories with every bite. Plus, that fiber isn't just filling up space; it's also fueling a healthy metabolism and keeping things running smoothly.

On the other hand, meat and animal products have a much higher caloric density. They lack water and fiber, so calorie for calorie, you end up with a smaller portion on your plate. It's like getting less bang for your buck, except we're talking about your calorie budget here. So, plants are your best pals if you want to feel full without tipping the scales.

One side effect of consuming fewer calories is that you might want to eat more often (which is fine if it's the right thing) but eat the wrong things, and you could experience weight gain.

Now, I'm not saying all plant foods are low in calories. Nuts and seeds, for instance, are pretty calorie-dense, but they're also rich in nutrients and healthy fats that are good for your heart and brain. The trick is to balance these with other, less calorie-dense foods like leafy greens and fresh fruits, stacking the deck (or, in this case, the plate) in favor of overall caloric moderation.

What's more, focusing on the caloric density of foods can transform your relationship with eating. It's not about stringent portion control or calorie counting that can take the joy out of meals. It's about embracing a way of eating where you can savor a cornucopia of foods without worrying about restricting yourself to tiny portions or battling constant hunger.

And here's a neat metabolic bonus: foods lower in caloric density typically require more energy to digest. This phenomenon, known as the thermic effect of food, means your body burns more calories processing these nutrient powerhouses. So not only are you ingesting fewer calories, but you're also using more energy to break those calories down. It's a win-win for your metabolism and your waistline.

When you fill your diet with plants, you're not just cutting calories; you're providing your body with all the essentials for peak performance. From vitamins and minerals to those incredible phytonutrients we talked about earlier, you're fueling up on the good stuff while keeping your calorie count in check without even trying.

So, when you're pondering how to manage your weight and supercharge your metabolism, remember that the plant kingdom has your back. A bounty of fresh produce, wholesome grains, and hearty legumes are waiting to nourish you.

By harnessing plants' power and lower caloric density, you can enjoy a satisfying, health-promoting diet that supports your weight management goals effortlessly. Trust me, your body will thank you for it!

As we move through our journey of understanding, let's keep in mind that the key is not to obsess over numbers but to focus on the quality and diversity of the food we eat.

Plant foods invite us into a world where we can eat abundantly, live healthily, and manage our weight naturally. It's a delicious approach to life that our bodies are designed to thrive on, and it's worth every bite.

The Role of Plants in Fat Loss

As you explore the path to a leaner self, it's essential to understand how plants contribute to fat loss. Unlike their meaty counterparts, plant-based foods have a secret weapon in this struggle: a lower caloric density. This means you can indulge in a larger volume of food while consuming fewer calories, making for a satisfied stomach without the guilt.

Eating your greens (reds and yellows!) is no short-lived diet trend. A lifestyle change brings a cascade of health benefits, including weight management. Plants are crammed with fiber, which doesn't just keep the digestive tract purring like a well-oiled machine; it helps control blood sugar levels and keeps you feeling full for longer. Thus, the urge to raid the snack drawer mid-afternoon starts to wane.

While we're on blood sugar, let's talk about the glycemic index. Natural plant-based foods often have a lower glycemic load, helping you avoid the spike-and-crash cycle from processed and high-sugar foods. Steady energy levels throughout the day mean you're less likely to reach for quick fixes high in sugar and fat.

Another plant-provided gem is the action of phytochemicals. These are powerful compounds that, among their numerous benefits, may boost metabolism and aid in breaking down fats more effectively. Drinking green tea can also help boost metabolism in some cases.

And when it comes to building muscle, don't think meat has the monopoly on protein. Plants can also pack a punch with their protein content, which is vital for maintaining and building lean muscle mass - the more muscle you have, the quicker your metabolism works, even at rest. This means your body becomes more efficient at burning calories.

But it's not just about what's in plants; it's also what's not. Typical plant-based diets are lower in saturated fat, which is often found in abundance in animal products. Less saturated fat in your system means your body can focus on burning stored fat rather than dealing with excess dietary fat.

However, you need to eat healthy meals on a consistent regular basis. If you have an unpredictable, irregular eating pattern (and your body doesn't know when it will eat next), you could be training it to store fat instead of burning it.

Now, let's talk about the weight of water – quite literally. Vegetables and fruits are high in water content, contributing to hydration, which is crucial for every cellular process in your body, including fat metabolism.

Often, adequate hydration can increase the number of calories you burn in a day. But you still need to drink a lot of water to stay hydrated - one crude method to consider is that if your urine is not clear, you are not drinking enough water.

It's also important to note the holistic approach to weight management through plant-based nutrition. While plants assist in reducing fat, they also enrich the body with essential vitamins and minerals for optimal health. It's a win-win scenario that bolsters your overall well-being while trimming the waistline.

Finally, embracing a variety of colorful plants looks great on your plate and ensures a broad spectrum of nutrients, each with its unique role in supporting metabolism and weight loss. With every bite, you're recruiting a small army to help battle against unhealthy fat accumulation.

Commit to incorporating more plants into your diet, and watch as they work their subtle magic on your body. Remember, it's not about denying yourself the foods you love but about finding plant-based alternatives that satisfy, nourish, and help you reach your weight loss goals.

Now, with all that fresh in your mind, let me give you the hard truth: Going vegan does not automatically mean you'll lose weight. It is true that eating a "whole-food, plant-based diet" is very likely going to help you lose weight - the fine print is in the catchphrase, "Whole Foods."

Many cookies, cakes, and breads are vegan, but consuming loads of carbohydrates (not healthy veggies) can contribute to weight gain. Your body does need carbohydrates, but healthy ones.

Sometimes, if a new vegan doesn't know what to eat or doesn't have time to cook, they might replace healthy whole foods with vegan junk food instead, which will have the opposite effect of losing weight. So remember to eat a whole-food, plant-based diet (the less processed, the better), and you should be good.

Another thing to remember (if you're trying to lose weight) is that the old adage is still valid, "You need to burn more calories than you consume to lose weight."

Chapter 9: Mental Wellbeing and Cognitive Functions

Moving beyond the physical, let's talk about what feeds the powerhouse behind it all – our brains. Connecting the dots between a plant-based diet and your mental well-being; it's crucial to understand how what we eat impacts our bodies and our thoughts, emotions, and cognitive sharpness.

Plants are nature's multivitamins, filled with compounds that keep our neural pathways firing effectively. Unlike their meaty counterparts, plant foods are rich in antioxidants, which combat oxidative stress – a villain in the story of cognitive decline.

This chapter delves into how embracing leafy greens, vibrant fruits, and hearty grains could benefit your waistline and be a blessing for your brain health.

Now, let's get personal for a moment. We've all had those days – feeling the brain fog, maybe a bit down in the dumps, or stressed out. It's perfectly human. But imagine having a secret weapon that helps regulate your mood and arm you against stress.

That's right, plants can be this hidden superpower. Foods such as avocados, nuts, and seeds aren't just tasty; they're packed with essential fatty acids that are key players in brain function and mood stabilization.

Carbs - whole ones, though, like oats and quinoa, are good for you. They support serotonin production, the feel-good neurotransmitter that keeps the blues at bay.

A plant-based diet encourages a symphony of these nutritional heroes to work in your favor, possibly reducing anxiety and boosting that feel-good vibe.

Now, chew on this idea: what if the road to sharper thinking, memory, and focus doesn't involve a fancy supplement or a challenging brain game but simply changing what's on your plate?

A diet high in plants is a treasure chest of phytonutrients and minerals that support cognitive functions for learning and memory. From the flavonoids in blueberries to the omega-3s in flaxseeds, these gifts from the plant world have been associated with decreased rates of cognitive decline. Plus, with plants, we're talking sustainable energy that keeps you alert and ready to tackle the tasks at hand.

So, when you're craving that mental edge, consider that a vibrant, plant-rich diet could be your faithful ally, helping you stay as sharp as a tack and feel mentally balanced.

Diet and Brain Health (Cognitive Memory Function)

As we venture further into the exploration of plant-based nutrition, let's pause and focus on a less-discussed yet incredibly important topic: the impact of your diet on brain health.

If the eyes are the window to the soul, then our diet might be the foundation upon which cognitive function is built. And guess what? Plants are crucial to unlocking a vibrant, sharp, and resilient mind. It's fascinating. The notion is that the foods we consume can mold our mental acuity.

Multiple studies have joined the chorus, emphasizing that a diet rich in fruits, vegetables, nuts, and seeds is associated with lower risks of cognitive decline and various neurodegenerative diseases. This isn't just a random finding; the compounds found abundantly in plants have brain-benefitting superpowers.

Let's talk antioxidants, the brain's defense squad against oxidative stress. Oxidative stress contributes to the aging process and can play a part in the development of conditions like Alzheimer's disease.

Plant foods are teeming with these heroic antioxidants, fighting a valiant battle against the rusting of our brain cells. It's as if each leafy green and berry is a miniature shield against cognitive decay.

Then there's inflammation, the silent enemy within that's linked not only to joint pain or heart trouble but also to mental malaise. A plant-based diet is replete with anti-inflammatory compounds that help keep the fires of inflammation at bay. By choosing plant foods over meat, you select the most natural form of inflammation fighters.

Let's remember fats. Omega-3 fatty acids (the good guys found in flaxseeds, chia seeds, and walnuts) are crucial for brain health. They're the building blocks for cell membranes and are indispensable for cognitive functions. Contrast this with the saturated fats from meat, which have the opposite effect, potentially clogging arteries and slowing down the body and the brain.

Now, consider fiber. Yep, fiber. It's not just for digestion. A high-fiber diet from plant sources does wonders for gut health. And a happy gut means a happy brain, thanks to the gut-brain axis.

This is where the conversation pivots to the microbiome, a community of friendly gut inhabitants that play a part in mood regulation and brain function. Feed them plant fibers, and they'll produce short-chain fatty acids, which are like love notes to your brain.

The brainpower of berries and the cognition-boosting brawn of broccoli are exceptional. The natural phytochemicals in these plants, which give them vivid colors and distinct flavors, are also neuroprotective. They're not just making your plate look pretty; they're safeguarding your brain's future.

Cognitive Problems: Possible Causes

On the flip side, have you ever considered how meat could affect your brain? Beyond the heart health talk, researchers have found associations between meat consumption and increased risk factors for cognitive issues. Saturated fats **and heavy metals** found in some fish, meats, and baked goods might be the culprits here, contributing to brain fog and other cognitive challenges.

Alzheimer's & Cognitive Memory Loss

Alzheimer's disease is a progressive neurological disorder that causes cognitive decline, memory loss, and changes in behavior, ultimately leading to severe impairment in daily functioning. It is the most common form of dementia.

It is characterized by the **accumulation of abnormal protein deposits** in the brain, which interfere with the normal functioning of brain cells and lead to their degeneration and death.

In baked goods, Sodium Aluminum Phosphate reacts with acidic ingredients such as cream of tartar or lemon juice to produce carbon dioxide gas, which helps dough or batter rise and become light and fluffy. This process is known as leavening and is essential for making baked goods like cakes, muffins, and pancakes.

While sodium aluminum phosphate is generally recognized as safe by regulatory authorities **when used in small quantities** in food products, there has been some controversy surrounding the safety of aluminum compounds in general.

Some studies have suggested a potential link between aluminum exposure and health issues such as Alzheimer's disease. Still, the evidence is inconclusive, and regulatory agencies like the Food and Drug

Administration (FDA) have deemed aluminum compounds safe for use in food when used within established limits.

What they don't tell you is that (like all heavy metals) **aluminum compounds are bio-accumulative**, which means they tend to store up in your fatty tissue - particularly around the brain.

Some studies have reported higher levels of aluminum in the brains of individuals with Alzheimer's disease compared to those without the disease. However, it's important to note that these findings do not necessarily prove causation, and the role of aluminum in the development of Alzheimer's disease remains a topic of debate among scientists.

One study published in 2017 (by Exley et al. in the Journal of Trace Elements in Medicine and Biology) reported elevated levels of aluminum in brain tissue samples from individuals with Alzheimer's disease compared to age-matched controls.

The researchers analyzed brain tissue samples using a specialized technique called fluorescence microscopy and found higher concentrations of aluminum in specific regions of the brain associated with Alzheimer's pathology.

Another study published in 2018 (by Mirza et al. in the Journal of Alzheimer's Disease) reported higher levels of aluminum in the fatty tissue (adipose tissue) of individuals with Alzheimer's disease compared to healthy controls.

The researchers collected adipose tissue samples from individuals undergoing surgery and measured aluminum levels using a technique called inductively coupled plasma mass spectrometry.

They found that individuals with Alzheimer's disease **had significantly higher levels of aluminum in their adipose tissue** compared to controls.

The overall scientific consensus is that the role of aluminum in Alzheimer's disease is still uncertain and requires further investigation.

While avoiding excessive aluminum exposure may be prudent as a precautionary measure, more research is needed to understand better the relationship between aluminum and Alzheimer's disease, cognitive memory loss, thinking functioning, and reasoning) and to determine whether reducing aluminum exposure could help prevent or treat the disease.

Explain That in English Please

All this means is that a sharp, alert, and emotionally stable mind isn't just a result of genetics or chance - it's deeply influenced by what you eat.

When brain cells are nurtured with plant-based goodness, they thrive, making a compelling case for a diet rooted in the earth's bounty. And this isn't just fluff and good feelings; it's backed by compelling scientific studies pointing to the cognitive casino jackpot, where plants are always the winning bet.

However, when you consume and collect a lot of "abnormal proteins" and "bio-accumulative heavy metals," take notice that you are not building a healthy brain.

So imagine this: a future where our mental span stretches long into our twilight years, where memories remain crisp, and where the brain fog that we've come to accept as 'just getting older' is no longer inevitable.

Holding the keys to such a future in our very hands is empowering whenever we choose what to eat. A plant-based diet is not just a choice for now; it's a commitment to a mentally rich life full of vivid thoughts and unfading memories.

Mood and Stress Regulation

Lifestyles today can be whirlwinds of tasks and responsibilities, leading to an epidemic of stress and mood disorders that can reduce our quality of life. But amidst this, there's a powerful, natural ally at our disposal - the food we put on our plates.

Our focus now turns to the profound impact of a plant-based diet on mood and stress regulation and how it supports mental well-being.

Let's cut to the chase - stress is a beast, and mood swings can make us feel like we're on a roller coaster. We've long known that diet has some role to play here, but only recently have we begun to understand how integral the connection is. Turning toward plants can provide unexpected but highly effective nourishment for our brains and moods.

For starters, a diet rich in whole plant foods is packed with vitamins, minerals, and antioxidants, which help protect brain cells from damage. These nutrients are good for our bodies, and they're fuel for our brains, too. Leafy greens, for instance, are rich in folate, which is crucial for mood regulation and preventing neurological deterioration. With their antioxidant punch, Berries can help manage inflammation, which is often a culprit in mood disorders.

And we can't talk about stress without addressing the BFF (Best Friend Forever) of the mental health world - B vitamins. Plants like nuts, seeds, and whole grains are little powerhouses of B vitamins, which have been shown to help reduce stress.

They're key players in synthesizing neurotransmitters that control mood and stress levels, like serotonin and dopamine. Also, the presence of fiber in plant foods helps in the slow release of glucose into your bloodstream, which means more steady energy levels and mood, unlike the crash and burn you might get from a meat-heavy, high-fat meal.

Omega-3 fatty acids are often praised for their role in cognitive function and mood stabilization. Flaxseeds, chia seeds, and walnuts, which are staples of a plant-based diet, provide ALA – a type of omega-3 that our bodies can convert to the brain-boosting EPA and DHA.

While you might've been told that fish is the go-to for omega-3s, plant-based sources are sustainable and don't come with the risk of mercury exposure that some seafood has.

Then there's magnesium, a mineral dubbed 'nature's relaxant.' Whole plants like spinach, pumpkin seeds, and black beans are bursting with it. Low levels of magnesium have been linked with an increase in anxiety and depression symptoms, so chomping down on magnesium-rich plants could be a ticket to a calmer, happier you.

Plants also support our gut health, which is a big deal because our gut is often termed the 'second brain.' An abundance of fiber from a plant-based diet supports a healthy gut microbiome, which produces about 95% of the body's serotonin. This neurotransmitter is a crucial regulator of mood, and guess what? It's primarily made in your gut, not your brain.

Adopting a plant-based diet encourages more than physical nourishment - it's about building resilience. With the complex synergy of phytonutrients and minerals, these foods help your body better cope with stress. The result? Fewer mood fluctuations and an overall sense of well-being that can feel like a breath of fresh air.

And let's not overlook the emotional and psychological advantages. Making conscious, compassionate food choices can have a positive impact on our self-esteem and outlook.

There's an empowering element to taking charge of your health and knowing that your choices are environmentally sustainable and kind to animals.

A famous musician named Paul McCartney once stated, "If slaughterhouses had glass walls, everyone would be vegetarian."

There is an incredible amount of violence and cruelty involved in the factory farming industries, which most people have no idea. This reminds me of another book you should read titled "World Peace Diet" (see Appendix C)

So, in closing, if stress is gnawing at your peace of mind or your mood feels like it's on a perpetual pendulum, consider reaching for greens over grilled meat.

Embrace the vibrancy of fruits, the satiety of legumes, the crunch of seeds, and the wholesomeness of whole grains. A plant-based diet isn't just a choice for the body; it's a boon for the brain. It's food designed for surviving and thriving - mind, body, and soul.

Chapter 10: Longevity and Disease Prevention

Imagine living in a world where triple-digit birthdays not only possibility but expected. This isn't just a fantasy. In certain pockets around the globe, known as Blue Zones, people are living longer than anywhere else on Earth. And guess what? Their diets are heavily plant-based.

We're talking about a lifestyle rich in fruits, vegetables, legumes, whole grains, and nuts. These foods are fuel and the building blocks of a long and vibrant life. These people are living longer and better. They have fewer chronic diseases, which means more years of good health, clarity of mind, and the ability to maintain an active lifestyle.

So what about the scary 'C' word? Cancer.

It's a concern that's touched many lives, but here's an empowering truth - your plate is your shield. Many plant foods are packed with phytonutrients that work like a team of bodyguards, providing an anti-cancer effect.

Cruciferous veggies like broccoli and Brussels sprouts, beans of all stripes, berries by the basketful - they're tasty, and they potentially deter cancer cells from setting up shop in your body. It's like an invisible armor, and the research backing this up is robust and growing.

By filling your diet with a variety of plant-based foods, you're taking an active role in your health narrative, reducing the risk of cancer with every bite. You're investing in your longevity bank account.

Let's not forget the other culprits of shortened lifespans: heart disease, diabetes, and stroke. They can often be traced back to lifestyle choices, with diet playing a critical role.

Switching to a plant-based diet can be like putting up a stop sign in the path of these diseases. The high fiber, rich antioxidants, and healthy fats inherent in plant-based foods contribute to smoother blood flow, balanced blood sugar, and reduced inflammation.

This kind of eating pattern adds years to life and life to years. With disease prevention as a delicious side effect of nutritious eating, what's not to love? Look at it this way: every plant-based meal is a step toward a longer, healthier life. Now that's what you call a tasty investment.

Blue Zones and Longevity Hotspots

So, you're curious about the secrets behind some of the longest-living populations on Earth, the so-called Blue Zones?

Well, in these longevity hotspots, where a significant number of individuals live past 100 years, diet plays a crucial role. And guess what? The common denominator across these regions is a heavy reliance on plant-based foods.

In short, Blue Zones are regions of the world where people are known to live significantly longer and healthier lives compared to the global average.

These areas have attracted attention from researchers and health enthusiasts seeking to understand the factors contributing to longevity and well-being. The concept of Blue Zones was popularized by National Geographic Fellow and journalist Dan Buettner, who identified and studied these regions.

These zones offer compelling evidence of how a diet rich in vegetables, fruits, grains, and legumes can contribute to an extended lifespan and a marked reduction in disease.

There are currently five recognized Blue Zones:

- **Ikaria, Greece**: Located in the Aegean Sea, Ikaria is known for its high concentration of centenarians (people who live to be 100 years or older). The residents of Ikaria enjoy a traditional Mediterranean diet rich in fruits, vegetables, olive oil, whole grains, and legumes. They also maintain an active lifestyle, engage in regular physical activity, and prioritize social connections and community involvement.

- **Okinawa, Japan**: Okinawa is an archipelago in southern Japan with one of the highest life expectancies in the world. The people of Okinawa follow a diet known as "Hara Hachi Bu," which emphasizes moderation, portion control, and a plant-based approach. Their diet includes plenty of vegetables, tofu, seaweed, and very small amounts of fish and meat. Additionally, Okinawans maintain strong social bonds, engage in lifelong learning, and practice stress-reducing activities such as meditation and tai chi.

- **Sardinia, Italy**: Sardinia is an island in the Mediterranean Sea with a high concentration of centenarians. The traditional Sardinian diet includes whole grains, beans, vegetables, fruits, nuts, olive oil, and some dairy products, as well as occasional consumption of meat and wine. Sardinians also lead active lifestyles, often working in agriculture or tending to their land well into old age. Strong family ties and a sense of belonging to a tight-knit community are also important aspects of life in Sardinia.

- **Nicoya Peninsula, Costa Rica**: The Nicoya Peninsula is a region of Costa Rica known for its high life expectancy and low rates of chronic disease. The diet of Nicoyans is based on locally grown fruits, vegetables, beans, rice, and corn, as well as occasional consumption of fish and meat. Physical activity is an integral part of daily life, with many Nicoyans engaging in farming, gardening, and other outdoor activities. Social connections and a sense of purpose are also important factors contributing to well-being in this region.

- **Loma Linda, California, USA**: Loma Linda is a community in Southern California with a large population of Seventh-day Adventists, a religious group known for promoting a health-conscious lifestyle. Adventists in Loma Linda follow a plant-based diet, abstaining from meat, fish, alcohol, and tobacco. They prioritize regular exercise, stress management, and spiritual well-being. Strong social networks and community support are also key aspects of life in Loma Linda.

In addition to these five recognized Blue Zones, there are other regions around the world with similar characteristics and longevity patterns.

The study of Blue Zones has provided valuable insights into the factors that contribute to long and healthy lives, including diet, lifestyle, social connections, and a sense of purpose and belonging. Incorporating Blue Zone lessons into our lives can help promote longevity, well-being, and vitality.

Digging deeper into the Blue Zones, we notice patterns in their eating habits.

They don't just eat plants; their diet focuses on whole, unprocessed foods. The vibrancy of fresh produce, the wholesomeness of grains, and the sustenance from legumes grace their plates daily. It's a stark contrast to the meat-heavy diets that are often linked to a plethora of health issues.

This plant-based approach nourishes and protects their bodies, acting like a shield against diseases that are all too common where animal-based foods dominate diets.

Now, let's address a critical aspect of these diets - protein. Even without meat, older people in Blue Zones obtain ample protein from plants.

They're living, robust proof that the myth of needing meat for protein is just that - a myth.

Legumes, nuts, and whole grains provide the essential amino acids their bodies require. This goes hand-in-hand with the evidence we've already touched upon regarding the power of plant proteins.

The Blue Zones aren't just about what's on the dinner table. There's a symbiotic relationship between their diet and lifestyle. The physical activity of gardening, walking to visit neighbors, or doing household chores helps to assimilate the nutrients from these plant-powered diets, creating a harmonious cycle of health and well-being. It's not a romance with gyms or marathons but rather an everyday, gentle integration of movement and purpose.

Just as important is the emphasis on social engagement and community. Eating isn't just for sustenance in these regions; it's a social event that reinforces community bonds.

The emotional and psychological health derived from strong social ties is critical to longevity. So, it's not only about what they eat, but also how they eat - with joy, in community, and without the overconsumption that's rampant in many cultures today.

But the most persuasive aspect, coming from these longevity hotspots, is the reduced incidence of chronic diseases.

In the Blue Zones, lower rates of heart disease, diabetes, obesity, and certain cancers are a testament to the power of their predominant plant-based diets. It makes you think: if a diet can offer such profound protective effects, isn't it worth considering? After all, we're talking about delicious, colorful, and versatile ingredients that tantalize the taste buds and add years to your life.

Think about the impact of such a diet on healthcare systems. These long-lived communities are living examples of how such a dietary pattern could drastically reduce the need for medical interventions for chronic conditions that plague many. Simple yet so profound, their way of life offers a blueprint for disease prevention that's built around plants, not pills.

The elders in these regions lead lives characterized by purpose, activity, and joy - factors that are intimately tied to their diet. They age gracefully, free from the common medications and interventions in their meat-consuming counterparts. Quality of life in later years is as important as quantity, and their plant-forward diets are at the heart of this high quality of life.

So, as you explore the concept of a plant-based diet for health and longevity, let the Blue Zones serve as a beacon. These populations are not just surviving; they're thriving. And while genetics and other factors might have their roles, it's crystal clear that diet is a cornerstone of their extraordinary longevity. It's not a tale of restriction but one of abundance – an abundance of health, vitality, and years.

The evidence is as ripe and ready as the fruit hanging from the trees in an Okinawan garden. What we eat matters, not just for our waistlines but for the timeline of our lives.

Before we transition into the role of plant diets in cancer prevention, let's take these lessons to heart. It's about a whole, plant-based diet, simplicity, community, and the joy of eating foods that love us back.

That's the secret behind the Blue Zones, and it's available to everyone – if only we choose to embrace it.

Cancer Prevention and Plant Diets

Continuing our exploration into the life-enhancing benefits of plant-based diets, let's delve into a critical area of disease prevention that has touched so many lives, often with heartbreaking effects: cancer.

The statistics can feel overwhelming; however, emerging research institutions have started to shed hopeful light on the potent protective effects of plant-based diets in the war against cancer.

The foods we put on our plates could be one of our strongest allies in this battle.

If you don't know exactly what it is, cancer is a complex group of diseases characterized by the uncontrolled growth and spread of abnormal cells in the body. These abnormal cells can invade and destroy surrounding healthy tissues, impairing the function of organs and leading to serious health complications.

Cancer can develop in almost any part of the body and can arise from various factors, including genetic mutations, environmental exposures, lifestyle choices, and infectious agents.

For starters, plants are packed with diverse nutrients that work together to strengthen our body's natural defenses.

Phytochemicals, the natural compounds found in fruits, vegetables, grains, and legumes, have been observed to help prevent cancer in many ways. They can help neutralize carcinogens, reduce inflammation, prompt cell repair, and even initiate the death of damaged cells, a process known as apoptosis.

Take antioxidants, for example; they're like the body's cleanup crew, sweeping up the free radicals that can lead to DNA damage and subsequent cancer development. A diet rich in plant-based foods provides a vast array of antioxidants, striking at the oxidative stress that can aid and abet carcinogenesis (the initiation of cancer formation).

Then there's fiber, the unsung hero in the nutrition world. It's abundant in plant-based diets, and while many people know it's good for digestion, its role in cancer prevention deserves spotlight attention. Fiber fermentation in the gut produces short-chain fatty acids with protective effects that resonate through the colon.

By promoting regular bowel movements, fiber helps ensure that potential carcinogens in the food we eat are excommunicated hastily from the body, reducing their contact time with the gut lining and decreasing the risk of colorectal cancer. In the next chapter, I will tell you a personal story about this type of cancer.

We can't ignore the importance of an appropriate body weight in reducing cancer risk; this is where a whole-food, plant-based diet excels. With lower calorie densities and high nutrient content, such diets help manage a healthy weight, thus reducing the cancer risk associated with obesity and overweight.

Shifting the focus to specific types of cancer, like breast and prostate, the evidence mounts. Diets high in fatty meat and dairy products have been linked to higher incidences of these hormone-responsive cancers.

Plant-based diets, low in fat and devoid of animal hormones, are emerging as a practical prevention strategy, helping to modulate the body's hormone levels and minimize risk.

Even after a cancer diagnosis, embracing plants can make a difference. Survivor stories often highlight a transition to plant-dominant eating. While anecdotal, they're backed by evidence illustrating how such dietary patterns can slow cancer progression and support the body during traditional treatment regimens.

Skeptics might point out that plants themselves contain naturally occurring compounds that can be considered carcinogenic. However, the dosage makes the poison, and the levels of these in a balanced plant-based diet are far below harmful; indeed, their presence is often counteracted by the symphony of beneficial nutrients also provided by plants.

Considering the emerging understanding of how certain plant compounds can influence gene expression, we're seeing that our food choices might play a role in 'turning off' certain genes predisposed to cancer.

The field of nutrigenomics is exploding, and it is here that the plant-based diet truly shines, offering hope that our forks might wield more power than we ever realized.

Lastly, let's not forget that adopting a plant-based diet isn't just an isolated strategy - it often comes with a constellation of other health-promoting behaviors like regular physical activity, not smoking, and minimizing alcohol consumption.

Together, these lifestyle choices create a synergy that can herald a significant reduction in cancer risk.

Embracing a plant-based diet is akin to cultivating a garden within, where the seeds of longevity and disease resistance can sprout and flourish.

The protective effects of plant nutrients against cancer are no mere coincidence; they're a compelling testament to the power of our dietary choices in shaping our health destiny.

As the saying goes, an apple a day might not just keep the doctor away, but it could be part of a larger dietary armor against one of modern medicine's greatest adversaries.

How to Prevent Cancer

If it wasn't clear from the above, let me give you some bullet points on how to prevent it.

I am not a doctor or physician, so don't construe this as medical advice. I'm just an average guy where this topic hit pretty close to home and caused me to dive deep into diet and nutrition research.

Preventing cancer involves adopting healthy lifestyle habits and minimizing exposure to known risk factors. Here are some strategies to help reduce the risk of developing cancer:

- **Maintain a Healthy Weight**: Being overweight or obese is associated with an increased risk of several types of cancer, including breast, colorectal, prostate, and endometrial cancer. Aim to achieve and maintain a healthy weight through a balanced diet and regular physical activity.

- **Eat a Healthy Diet**: Consume a diet rich in fruits, vegetables, whole grains, and legumes, which are high in vitamins, minerals, fiber, and phytochemicals that have been shown to have protective effects against cancer. Eliminate intake of processed foods, meats, excess sugary foods, and refined carbohydrates.

- **Be Physically Active**: Physical activity can help reduce the risk of developing several types of cancer, including breast, colon, and prostate cancer so try to squeeze in some moderate to vigorous physical activity for about 30 minutes a day on a regular basis.

- **Avoid Tobacco**: Tobacco use is a leading cause of many types of cancer, including lung, mouth, throat, esophageal, and bladder cancer. Avoid smoking cigarettes, cigars, and pipes, and avoid exposure to secondhand smoke.

- **Limit Alcohol Consumption**: Excessive alcohol consumption is linked to an increased risk of several types of cancer, including breast, liver, colorectal, and esophageal cancer. Limit alcohol intake to below moderate levels, which is defined as up to one drink per day for women and up to two drinks per day for men. For me personally, I stopped drinking alcohol completely 25 years ago.

- **Protect Against Sun Exposure**: Protect your skin from the harmful effects of ultraviolet (UV) radiation by wearing sunscreen with a high SPF, seeking shade, wearing protective clothing, and avoiding outdoor activities during peak sun hours.

- **Get Screened**: Participate in recommended cancer screening tests and screenings for early detection of cancer, such as mammograms for breast cancer, Pap tests for cervical cancer, colonoscopies for colorectal cancer, and prostate-specific antigen (PSA) tests for prostate cancer. Early detection can greatly improve the chances of successful treatment and survival

Adopting these healthy lifestyle habits and minimizing exposure to known risk factors can help reduce your risk of developing cancer and promote overall health and well-being. Regular communication with your healthcare provider can help you make informed decisions about your health and reduce your risk of cancer.

Chapter 11: Navigating Social and Cultural Norms

As you embrace a plant-based diet, you might find yourself at a social event, staring at a buffet loaded with meat-heavy dishes, feeling like a lone plant amidst a field of grazing animals. That's when it hits: the probing glances, the raised eyebrows, the hushed questions. "No meat for you?"

A wave of realization flows over you; food is more than just sustenance; it's a cultural handshake, a social glue.

Adjusting to this new way of eating means rethinking not just what's on your plate but how you relate to those traditional, meat-focused norms that are deeply embedded in our social fabric.

Let's face it: Food choices can be personal, but they're also incredibly public. Whether it's family dinners, holiday feasts, or workplace lunches, what we eat often becomes a focal point of discussion and, sometimes, contention.

But here's the thing: navigating these complex waters doesn't have to leave you stranded. Being plant-based in a meat-centered world is a chance to showcase resilience, creativity, and commitment to personal health and ethical values.

While it's true that it can be daunting to field the never-ending 'where do you get your protein' interrogation, view these moments as opportunities.

Opportunities to share facts about plant-based nutrition, dispel myths, and maybe even intrigue Aunt Mary so much that she tries a spoonful of your vegan cheese cake. Think of it this way - you're not just eating differently, you're an ambassador for a healthier life and a more sustainable world.

Go on and savor your vibrant, vegetable-rich plate at that next potluck. Chances are you'll catch curious glances, followed by intrigued questions. Use these inquiries to your advantage, educate through example, and remember that cultural tides are shifting every day.

Around the world, there are pockets and traditions that celebrate plant-based eating - not as a trend, but as a part of their rich heritage. It's about embracing those roots and even discovering new plant-based celebrations.

The key is to stay true to your values while being understanding and patient with others. After all, once they see your energy and how you're thriving, they just might be tempted to dip their fork into the plant-based world too.

Dealing with Dietary Peer Pressure

Navigating the social waters while maintaining a plant-based diet can sometimes feel like swimming against the current.

The aroma of barbecue at family gatherings, the steaming pepperoni pizzas at work events, and the ever-present "Why aren't you eating meat?" question are part of the dietary peer pressure package.

Here, let's explore why a plant-based diet aligns with optimal health and how to manage the choppy waters of social norms and expectations.

First, let's appreciate that maintaining a diet (off the beaten path) requires gumption and self-assurance. The pressure to conform is real and can be overwhelming at times.

When you're faced with questioning glances and weird looks as you load your plate with veggies, it's important to remember your 'why.'

You must have a strong reason for doing this, or you probably won't stay with it (because friends and family sometimes have a way of knocking us out of the box). You will need to figure out what "your reason" is, but it was the undeniable health benefits for me.

My father ate a terrible, fatty, meat-rich diet all his life, and he died from colon cancer at age 46. A few years later, when I was almost age 30, I decided I didn't want to go out like that and die in my 40s from heart disease, stroke, or cancer.

Keep "Your Reason Why" at the forefront of your mind.

Your conviction can be just as contagious as the social pressure you're facing. Once you go down this amazing adventure of exploration into fantastic foods, related books, and plant-based diet documentaries (see Appendix C), your life will drastically change for the better and give you excitement to keep you going when the going gets tough.

Moreover, you're not just adopting a diet but embracing a lifestyle. When friends and family press you with their concerns (where do you get your protein?), for example - use these moments as opportunities to educate them. Many need to realize that plants can be excellent sources of all essential amino acids without the baggage of cholesterol and high saturated fat in meat.

Always remember that while it's okay to share knowledge, it's equally important to do so without appearing judgmental.

People get defensive if they feel attacked about their food choices. Be compassionate and show understanding because everyone's on their unique journey; many are a step behind yours.

Practice polite firmness when declining non-plant-based options. A simple statement like "No thank you, I do better on plants" can affirm your position without inciting a debate. Remember, you're not just saying no to a dish; you're saying yes to the health you cherish and yes to the values that guide you.

Diplomacy is very important for those trickier situations, like a grandma who can't understand why you won't eat her famous meatloaf.

Acknowledge the love behind the offering - "I know you made this with care, and I appreciate it," then gently explain that you're making choices that are right for your body.

Often, it's not about the food but the connection it symbolizes; let your loved ones know you can still share in the togetherness with alternative dishes.

When dining out, it's helpful to look up the menu beforehand and decide what you can eat. If your friends choose a steakhouse, most will have a vegetarian option, or you could choose a salad and a side. Or better yet, take the lead and suggest a spot known for its great plant-based options. It can be an eye-opening experience for your meat-loving friends.

There will be moments of discomfort but also moments of immense pride. Stand your ground, and you may inspire someone else to consider why you've made your choices. Your journey can influence others in the most unexpected ways, even if it just starts with curiosity about your bean chili that smells fantastic.

Don't be surprised if some social circles begin to embrace your dietary choices. Good friends will support your journey and might even get excited to try new plant-based recipes at your next potluck.

Some of your friends might also ridicule you. My best friend of 30 years gave me lots of criticism for 20 years about my vegetarian diet every time we tried to find a place to have lunch, which was usually 4-5 times a month. Then, a few years ago (after some personal reasons), he called me out of the blue and asked for suggestions because he was considering to give a plant-based diet a try and start making better choices about what he was eating - so you just never know where those seeds will sprout.

Change can start with one person's plate - yours, and always remember what Mahatma Gandhi said, "Be the change that you wish to see in the world."

It's important to remember that most Americans (and Europeans) have been indoctrinated into mainly eating meat for a very long time. Some of our fondest memories are around mealtimes with cookouts and social gatherings around food, so when you confront these feelings and emotions with facts, logic, and reason - those feelings and memories can often be met with contempt and ridicule.

Lastly, there's no need to face this alone. Connect with plant-based groups, online communities, or friends who share your dietary values. Here, you'll find support, understanding, and a treasure trove of experience dealing with the pressures you face. You can exchange stories, tips, and dishes that make staying true to your plant-based lifestyle manageable and enjoyable.

Overall, dealing with dietary peer pressure exercises patience, persistence, and poise.

As you skillfully navigate these social dynamics, armed with information and a heart full of reasons, you might find that the path becomes less resistant over time.

Feasting on your greens amidst the carnivores doesn't just bolster your health; it might also plant seeds of health consciousness in those around you. That's a win-win in any social setting.

Plant-Based Traditions Around the World

Digging deeper into social and cultural norms, let's turn our attention to the vibrant tapestry of plant-based traditions across the globe.

It's fascinating how different cultures have thrived on diets rich in fruits, vegetables, legumes, and grains long before the wave of modern science and health advocacy. These traditions offer us a window into a world where eating plant-based is a way of life seamlessly woven into the cultural fabric.

Asia

In many Asian cultures, for instance, the symbol of rice in meals can't be overlooked. It's a staple and a sacred element, often accompanied by a spectrum of plant-based side dishes like kimchi, seasoned vegetables, and tofu. Simplicity and balance are vital principles, reflecting a more profound philosophy that believes in nourishing body and soul.

As a matter of fact, one book you might want to read is "The China Study" by Dr. T. Colin Campbell and Thomas M. Campbell II. This book results from a 20-year study conducted in China, where the authors examined the dietary habits and health outcomes of rural Chinese populations compared to those in the United States and other Western countries.

The book explores the relationship between diet and health, mainly focusing on the impact of nutrition on chronic diseases such as cancer, heart disease, diabetes, and obesity.

Mediterranean

Then we journey to the Mediterranean, where olive oil dances in almost every dish, and the plant kingdom holds the court. From the sun-soaked tomatoes to the earthy legumes, the colors and flavors tell stories of longevity and zest for life.

The Mediterranean diet has made headlines for its heart-healthy benefits, advocating for moderate but predominantly plant-based eating patterns crowned with occasional red wine.

The overall health of people in the Mediterranean region is often considered relatively good compared to many other parts of the world. This observation is frequently attributed to the dietary and lifestyle patterns characteristic of the Mediterranean region, which have been associated with numerous health benefits.

The Mediterranean diet is also associated with psychological well-being, including improved mood, reduced risk of depression, and better overall quality of life. The traditional Mediterranean diet is a model for promoting health and wellness through dietary choices that prioritize whole, nutrient-dense foods and emphasize a balanced, enjoyable approach to eating.

Middle East

Let's remember the heart of Middle Eastern cuisine, where dishes like hummus, falafel, and tabbouleh star as plant-based delights, reflecting an age-old reliance on chickpeas, lentils, and fresh herbs. The abundance of spices and various textures create a culinary experience that delights the senses while filling the stomach with fibrous, nutrient-rich foods.

Overall, the Middle Eastern diet is characterized by a diverse array of flavorful and nutritious foods, emphasizing whole grains, fruits, vegetables, legumes, nuts, and olive oil. It reflects the culinary traditions and cultural heritage of the region while providing a balanced and healthful approach to eating.

Africa

In West Africa, the practice of centering meals around grains and tubers (like millet, sorghum, and yams) combined with a symphony of greens and beans demonstrates a reliance on Earth's offerings that dates back centuries. This cuisine doesn't just fuel the body; it sings the praises of the plants that sustain daily life and cultural identity.

In East Africa, my all-time favorite is Ethiopian food. If you happen to have authentic Ethiopian cuisine in your town, you must try the traditional vegetarian combo platter, known as "ye'tsom beyaynetu," which is a colorful and flavorful assortment of vegetarian dishes that showcase the rich culinary heritage of Ethiopia.

I will explain this one in detail because it is a dish you should not pass up.

Ye'tsom beyaynetu typically consists of various vegetarian dishes, each offering a unique blend of flavors, textures, and spices. Typical dishes included in the platter may vary but often include lentil stew (misir wot), split pea stew (kik alicha), chickpea stew (shiro wot), cabbage and carrot stew (tikil gomen), spicy collard greens (gomen), and stewed potatoes (dinich wot).

Each dish is prepared separately, with a base of onions, garlic, and spices sautéed in oil or Ethiopian butter (niter kibbeh). Lentils, split peas, chickpeas, vegetables, and other ingredients are added to the pot and cooked until tender, allowing the flavors to meld together and the sauces to thicken to a rich and flavorful consistency. The original niter kibbeh butter base is derived from dairy and is not vegan, but some restaurants can make it vegan.

The vegetarian dishes are arranged on a large platter, each occupying a separate section. The vibrant colors of the various stews and vegetables create an eye-catching display, inviting diners to indulge in a feast for both the eyes and the palate. The platter is often garnished with sprigs of fresh herbs and served with injera, a sourdough flatbread made from teff flour.

Ye'tsom beyaynetu is typically enjoyed family-style, with diners gathering around the platter and using torn pieces of injera to scoop up bites of the various dishes. In Ethiopian culture, sharing food in this communal manner symbolizes hospitality, togetherness, and camaraderie.

The vegetarian dishes in Ye'tsom Beyaynetu are known for their bold and aromatic flavors, which are achieved through the careful layering of spices such as berbere, turmeric, ginger, and garlic. Each dish offers a unique balance of heat, sweetness, and savory richness, creating a harmonious and satisfying dining experience.

Ye'tsom beyaynetu is a delicious and nutritious meal and a celebration of Ethiopia's diverse culinary traditions and the abundance of plant-based ingredients available in the region. It is enjoyed by vegetarians and meat-eaters alike, highlighting the versatility and appeal of Ethiopian cuisine.

India

A tour of Indian subcontinent cuisine reveals a dazzling array of vegetarian dishes, where legumes and vegetables are spiced to perfection, showcasing a historic and deeply held respect for life in all forms. With their rich use of lentils, veggies, and rice, Indian meals illustrate a time-honored tradition that's both nutrient-dense and steeped in spiritual significance.

The fantastic food from Indian Cuisine is another personal favorite of mine, so I need to go into detail about this one, too. The Indian diet in Asia, often called the Indian subcontinent, is incredibly diverse and influenced by a rich tapestry of cultures, traditions, and regional cuisines.

Many of the Indian population follow a vegetarian diet for cultural, religious, and philosophical reasons. Vegetarianism has deep roots in Indian culture, with many traditional dishes featuring a wide variety of vegetables, legumes, lentils, grains, and some dairy.

Indian Cuisine is renowned for its bold and aromatic flavors, achieved through a wide range of spices and herbs. Common spices include cumin, coriander, turmeric, cardamom, cinnamon, cloves, and chili peppers. These spices add depth of flavor and provide numerous health benefits.

The Indian subcontinent is home to a vast array of regional cuisines, each with unique ingredients, cooking techniques, and flavor profiles.

North Indian Cuisine is characterized by rich, creamy curries, flatbreads like naan and roti, and tandoori dishes cooked in a clay oven. South Indian Cuisine, on the other hand, features rice-based dishes like dosas and idlis, as well as spicy curries made with coconut milk and tamarind.

Rice and wheat are the two main staple foods in the Indian diet, with rice predominant in South India and wheat in North India. These grains are typically served alongside various lentils, beans, and vegetables, forming the basis of many traditional meals.

India is famous for its vibrant street food culture, with bustling markets and roadside stalls offering a wide range of snacks and small bites. Popular street foods include chaat (savory snacks), samosas, pakoras, vada pav (potato fritter sandwich), and various dosas and parathas.

Indian Cuisine features a plethora of sweet treats and desserts, often made with ingredients like milk, sugar, ghee (clarified butter), nuts, and spices. Popular desserts include gulab jamun, rasgulla, jalebi, kheer (rice pudding), and various types of halwa (sweet confections).

Concerning health, Ayurveda, the ancient system of traditional medicine from India, plays a significant role in shaping dietary practices and food choices. Ayurvedic principles emphasize the importance of balancing different tastes (sweet, sour, salty, bitter, pungent, and astringent) in meals to promote health and well-being.

Overall, the Indian diet in Asia is characterized by its diversity, flavorfulness, and emphasis on fresh, seasonal ingredients. It reflects a deep connection to culinary traditions, cultural heritage, and health and wellness principles passed down through generations.

Europe

Even in European countries, where meat has often featured prominently in the diet, there's a strong undercurrent of plant-based eating. From the potato-and-cabbage-heavy dishes of Eastern Europe to the vegetable gardens that dot Italian landscapes, there's an acknowledgment of the importance of plants on the plate for health and satisfaction.

Vegetarian cuisine here has gained popularity in recent years, and numerous delicious vegetarian dishes are enjoyed across the continent. Here are some favorite vegetarian foods in Europe:

- Caprese Salad (**Italy**): A classic Italian salad made with fresh tomatoes, mozzarella cheese, basil leaves, olive oil, balsamic vinegar, salt, and pepper. It's a simple yet flavorful dish that highlights the vibrant flavors of Mediterranean ingredients.

- Greek Salad (**Greece**): A traditional Greek salad, also known as Horiatiki, typically consists of fresh tomatoes, cucumbers, red onions, bell peppers, olives, and feta cheese, dressed with olive oil, lemon juice, salt, and oregano. It's a refreshing and nutritious dish that showcases the flavors of Greek cuisine.

- Ratatouille (**France**): A classic French vegetable stew made with eggplant, zucchini, bell peppers, tomatoes, onions, garlic, and herbs such as thyme, basil, and parsley. It's a comforting and flavorful dish that can be served as a main course or side dish.

- Spanakopita (**Greece**): A traditional Greek savory pastry made with layers of phyllo dough filled with a mixture of spinach, feta cheese, onions, garlic, and herbs. It's a popular appetizer or snack that's both satisfying and delicious.

- Falafel (**Middle East**): While not originally European, falafel has become a favorite vegetarian street food in many European countries. These deep-fried balls or patties made from ground chickpeas or fava beans are typically served in pita bread with salad, tahini sauce, and pickles.

- Vegetarian Paella (**Spain**): A meatless version of the classic Spanish rice dish, paella, made with saffron-infused rice, vegetables such as bell peppers, tomatoes, peas, and artichokes, and flavored with garlic, paprika, and other spices. It's a colorful and flavorful dish that's perfect for sharing.

- Vegetarian Moussaka (**Greece**): A Greek casserole dish made with layers of eggplant, potatoes, and a hearty tomato sauce, topped with a creamy béchamel sauce and baked until golden and bubbly. It's a comforting and satisfying dish that's perfect for special occasions.

- Vegetarian Shepherd's Pie (**United Kingdom/Ireland**): A meatless version of the classic shepherd's pie, made with a filling of mixed vegetables such as carrots, peas, corn, and onions, topped with mashed potatoes and baked until golden and crispy. It's a hearty and comforting dish that's perfect for cold weather.

These are just a few examples of favorite vegetarian foods enjoyed in Europe. With its diverse culinary traditions and emphasis on fresh, seasonal ingredients, Europe offers a wide variety of delicious vegetarian dishes to suit every taste preference.

Native American

Lastly, in my home country, the indigenous peoples of the Americas embraced the power of plant-based eating. The "three sisters" (corn, beans, and squash) were not only nutritional staples but also a model of sustainability and regenerative agriculture. They understood that the health of the land was directly tied to personal and community well-being.

Native American cuisine is diverse and varies greatly among different tribes and regions across North America. Here are a few examples of favorite traditional Native American dishes:

- Fry bread is a beloved staple in many Native American communities. It is a versatile dish that can be served in various ways, including plain, topped with sweet or savory ingredients, or used as a base for dishes like Indian tacos.

- Three Sisters Stew is a traditional dish incorporates three staple crops of many Native American cultures: corn, beans, and squash. The three ingredients are combined with other vegetables, herbs, and sometimes meat to create a hearty and nutritious stew.

- Wild rice Casserole is a traditional food of many Native American tribes, particularly those in the Great Lakes region. It is often cooked with vegetables, herbs, and sometimes meat or fish to make a flavorful and nourishing casserole dish.

- Wojapi is a traditional berry sauce made from fresh or dried berries, water, and sometimes sweeteners like honey or maple syrup. It is often served as a topping for fry bread, pancakes, or other traditional foods.

These are just a few examples of favorite traditional Native American dishes, and there are many more delicious and culturally significant foods enjoyed by Indigenous communities across North America.

Summary

The common thread in all these traditions is the celebration of plants, not only as food but as life-giving, culture-shaping forces. Clearly, plant-based eating isn't merely a passing fad but has deep roots in our collective history. These practices show us that a plant-rich diet is viable, vibrant, delicious, and integrally aligned with human health.

As we consider these rich traditions, it becomes evident that the pull toward meat-centered diets in modern times isn't just a deviation from what's natural for our bodies; it's a move away from some of humanity's most nurturing and sustainable food practices.

Re-embracing plant-based diets can reconnect us with our history and guide us toward a healthier future.

In conclusion, these global plant-based traditions are enticing and inspirational. They help us navigate the often tricky waters of dietary changes, showing us that we're not alone - it's a path well-trodden with proven benefits for health and longevity.

By learning from these cultures, we can cultivate a richer, more rounded perspective on nourishing ourselves and respecting the planet, one meal at a time.

Taking the Leap - Transitioning to Plant-Based Eating

Now that we've navigated the choppy waters of social expectations and cultural traditions, it's time to wade into the refreshing stream of plant-based eating.

If the journey you've read through so far feels like it's resonating somewhere deep within, you might be ready to embrace this life-enhancing change.

Transitioning to a plant-based diet isn't about turning your back on centuries of culinary tradition but rather, rediscovering the rich bounty the plant kingdom has been offering. This journey is about liberation - a joyous adventure into renewed health, vibrant energy, and a sense of alignment with your values and the environment.

Begin with the staples; vegetables, fruits, whole grains, legumes, nuts, and seeds are your new best friends. Like any friendship, getting to know their likes and dislikes will take time. In other words, the preparation methods and pairings that best suit your palette might take some adjustment.

Starting with small changes makes the process less overwhelming; swap out that chunk of beef in your chili for beans or try a frozen entree in the meatless section at the grocery store. Go at your own pace, and remember, every meatless meal is a win for your health and the planet.

Speaking of the planet, did you know that you're effectively reducing your carbon footprint by going plant-based? It's like doing an environmental good deed with every meal.

Take a look at some of these scary environmental facts regarding the consumption of animals:

- Factory farming is a significant contributor to greenhouse gas emissions, particularly methane and nitrous oxide. Methane is produced by enteric fermentation in livestock, while nitrous oxide emissions result from manure management practices. Overall, livestock farming is estimated to contribute around 14.5% of global greenhouse gas emissions, according to the Food and Agriculture Organization of the United Nations.

- Factory farming requires extensive land for grazing, feed production, and animal housing. This can lead to deforestation, habitat destruction, loss of biodiversity, and soil degradation, particularly in regions where forests are cleared for agricultural expansion.

- Factory farming generates large quantities of animal waste, which can contaminate water sources through runoff and leaching, leading to water pollution and eutrophication (excessive toxins) that run off to a body of water, causing death to aquatic life from lack of oxygen. This excess of chemicals and antibiotics used in animal agriculture can further exacerbate water quality issues.

Building a plant-centered plate is both an art and a science. Picture your plate as a canvas, every hue of vegetable and grain a brush stroke that leads to a masterpiece of nutritional balance.

Focus on variety to ensure you're getting all the essential nutrients. A chorus of colorful veggies offers vitamins and antioxidants, whole grains bring the hearty satisfaction of fiber, and a sprinkle of nuts adds that delightful crunch and healthy fats.

And let's remember the culinary adventures awaiting in the world of spices and herbs; they're the secret to turning simple plant ingredients into gourmet experiences. You're not just nibbling on greens; you're indulging in a greens goddess salad adorned with an irresistible tahini dressing.

With each meal, celebrate the change you're making; your body, mind, and generations will thank you.

Beginning with Small Changes

Embarking on a journey to transform your eating habits can seem daunting at first glance.

You might envision spending a lot of money to completely overhaul your pantry and waste all that, or worry about giving up your favorite food, cold turkey. However, the secret to seamlessly shifting towards plant-based eating starts with small, manageable changes.

Begin with integrating more plant-based options into your meals, one dish at a time.

The next time you go grocery shopping, buy plant-based butter, vegan mayo, and almond milk to start with. If you pass through the frozen section, several plant-based alternatives exist in the ready-made frozen area. Even though they are processed with excess salts and preservatives, they might still make for good 'transition food' as you slowly switch to a whole-food, plant-based diet.

For me personally, when I first went vegetarian 26 years ago, I made a decision to do it and cut out most meats 'cold turkey' (pun intended) right away.

I continued to eat some fish and things with butter and cheese on them, but for the most part, I almost eliminated all meats from the start. That was easier for me, but for others, they may have to start slower.

For example, when I had to grab fast food, I would order a "burger - minus the patty" or a bean burrito instead of a beef one. It seemed odd initially, but the more I did that, the easier it was.

Let's start slow if you're not quite ready to go 'cold turkey.'

Visualize your typical dinner plate. Rather than replacing your main course with a plant-based alternative outright, begin by increasing the portion of vegetables and sneak some spinach into your lasagna.

When you have a bit more time on the weekends, instead of making an omelet, Google a plant-based recipe for tofu scramble! That is one of my favorites; I think you'll love that one.

If you plan to make pasta or spaghetti tonight, stop at the grocery store on the way home and visit the plant-based frozen section for some meatless meatballs or 'meatless crumbles' to add.

It's these subtle additions that can make significant health improvements without overwhelming your palate, your brain, or your routine.

Next, take a look at snacks - a perfect opportunity to introduce whole foods like fruit, nuts, and seeds instead of chips, junk food, or candy.

These natural goodies are not just filling; they're packed with nutrients and are simple to incorporate. Swap out chips for carrot sticks or that candy bar for a handful of almonds. The goal is to make these swaps feel as effortless as possible, building a foundation for more significant changes down the road.

Instead of cow's milk, use plant-based alternatives such as almond, soy, or oat milk in your cereal or coffee. These substitutes come in various flavors and can be a delightful taste exploration. You might be surprised at how creamy and satisfying these plant-based options can be, and your heart will thank you for the switch.

Speaking of exploration, spices and herbs are your best friends. They can transform any plant-based ingredient into a savory dish that rivals any meat-based counterpart. A sprinkle of cumin on roasted chickpeas, some basil on tomato slices, or a dash of cinnamon on sweet potatoes can elevate your meals to new levels of deliciousness, making the transition more about discovery than deprivation.

Furthermore, start incorporating whole grains, like quinoa, brown rice, or barley, into your meals. Aromatic and full of fiber, they satisfy a full belly and long-lasting energy without the sluggishness often accompanying processed grains. They harmonize beautifully with vegetables and legumes, creating a hearty base for many dishes.

Week by week, aim to reduce your meat portions while increasing your legumes, grains, and greens.

This adventure is all about finding new foods to love. Soon enough, meatless Mondays and taco Tuesdays (with meatless crumbles) could evolve into a more regular occurrence, leading to a newfound appreciation for meat-free meals that satisfy taste buds and nutritional needs.

And remember breakfast - it's an ideal meal to blend in more plants.

Start your day with a smoothie packed with fruits (see Appendix A), a splash of plant milk, and a handful of greens like spinach or kale. It's a nutritious, energizing way to greet the morning, and it can carry over the benefits of plant-based eating into the rest of your day.

Lastly, remember this isn't an all-or-nothing deal. Every bit of plant-based goodness adds up. Reducing meat consumption and increasing your intake of whole foods has substantial benefits for your health, and each meal is an opportunity to make a choice that supports well-being.

Be kind to yourself during this transition, allowing flexibility and patience as your taste buds and habits adjust naturally over time.

If you go 'cold-turkey' into a plant-based diet and lifestyle, be warned that it will take your body about two weeks to adjust and your taste buds to change from what you've been used to. I encourage you to stay the course for at least a month for the transition - don't give up; you can do it!

Taking small steps is a sustainable and enjoyable route to a plant-based diet. Before you know it, these incremental adjustments will lead to a substantial transformation in your health and your outlook on food.

As these habits settle in, you'll find the confidence to continue expanding your plant-based horizons, crafting a diet that's better for you and the planet.

Building a Plant-Centered Plate

Imagine crafting an edible mosaic rich in colors, textures, and nutrients; this is what building a plant-centered plate is all about.

It's more than removing animal products and filling the void with beige, less inspiring food. It's an adventure in flavors, a daily tour of the richness that nature can offer on your very plate.

Focusing on plants means celebrating the immense variety they bring to the table. The base of your plate should come from whole grains like brown rice, quinoa, barley, or farro - these hearty anchors make a meal satisfying. They're like dependable friends who never let you down, providing lasting energy thanks to their complex carbohydrates and fibers.

Around this base, we weave the vibrant threads of raw and cooked vegetables to provide diverse textures and flavors.

Greens like spinach, kale, and chard can be sautéed or tossed fresh into salads, while bell peppers, broccoli, and zucchini add crunch and color when roasted or stir-fried. It's a montage of nature's finest offerings, diverse enough to excite the palate and packed with vitamins and minerals.

Legumes then make their entrance. Think lentils, chickpeas, and black beans, which are the muscle of the plant world with their robust protein. When prepared with aromatic herbs and spices, they transform into the stars of your plate, capable of winning over the most skeptical taste buds.

And what's a plate without the accents: The nuts and seeds sprinkled on top for an extra dose of omega-3s, protein, and that satisfying crunch. Whether it's almond slivers over a bed of green beans or a sprinkle of sunflower seeds on your morning oatmeal, these little jewels bring great joy and nutrition.

Let's remember the fruit, nature's candy. It can brighten a breakfast or serve as a perfect sweet ending to your meal, with no added sugars. Plus, the antioxidants and fiber in fruits do wonders for your body from the inside out.

The beauty of building a plant-centered plate is that you don't just cater to your health; you also engage your senses. It's a visual feast as much as a nutritional one. And it's about variety; you don't need to eat the same old salad daily.

There are thousands of edible plants worldwide, each with unique flavors, textures, and nutrients. It's an incredible opportunity to be creative, explore, and nourish yourself thoroughly.

And if the thought of completely revamping your meals seems daunting, don't sweat it. It's about evolution, not revolution.

Start by making one plant-based meal a day and progress from there. Or take a beloved dish and twist it to be plant-forward: bolognese sauce with lentils, perhaps, or a hearty vegetable stew.

The aim is to reach a point where plants are the stars of your plate, not just the supporting cast. Switching to plant-based meals isn't about denial or rigid dieting; it's about reimagining how we eat to energize, protect, and rejuvenate our bodies.

And guess what? It may just be the most delicious decision you'll ever make.

Remember, your plate is your canvas, and you're the artist. There's no right or wrong way to paint it, as long as it's rich with plants. Get adventurous, taste new flavors, mix and match colors and textures, and watch as your health (and taste buds) thank you for it.

The Future is Green - A Vision for Health and Environment

So, we've ventured through the vast plains of nutrition, debunking myths and unearthing the bounty that is a plant-based diet.

Let's plant our feet firmly in the present and gaze into the horizon. The future we envision is vibrant, bursting with vitality for our physical well-being and our precious planet. A tapestry where each thread of choice we make weaves together a narrative of harmony and sustainability.

Imagine a world where our collective health is not a commodity but a commonwealth, where the food on our plates is not only a feast for our taste buds but also nourishment for our souls and solace for the environment.

Let's dream, for a moment, of a not-so-distant future where plant-based diets are the norm rather than the exception - a future where the life-giving force of whole, unprocessed foods curbs chronic diseases.

Compassion can be our compass, leading us towards dietary choices that respect our bodies and every creature sharing this planet with us.

A green future is also a kind one, where we no longer rely on the suffering of other beings for our sustenance. We've learned together that every morsel of plant-derived goodness supports a system free from the confinement and exploitation inherent in meat production.

As we stand at this crossroads, the footprint we leave behind becomes clear. A meat-centered diet not only treads heavily on our health but also on the ecosystems we inhabit.

By choosing a plant-based diet, we opt for the path with the lightest touch, preserving resources, nurturing biodiversity, and breathing life back into our soil and water. Let's embrace this green path that promises a future where humans and nature can thrive in mutual respect.

And let's remember the taste - the boundless array of textures and flavors the plant kingdom offers. There's a universe of grains, legumes, nuts, seeds, fruits, and vegetables waiting to be discovered.

Culinary creativity has no bounds when earthly gardens become our palette. A green future is flavorful, where the joy of eating is rediscovered and redefined.

Supporting this vision is a body of evidence, growing and showing without a shadow of a doubt that plant-based diets are a means to a healthy and hearty life.

It's about unlocking the potent combination of macro and micronutrients that put our well-being on an upward trajectory. From the sleek speed of athletes powered by plant protein to the gentle elders in Blue Zones, longevity is intricately woven into this green vision.

But how do we navigate this transition? It's all about small, purposeful changes that accumulate and make a significant impact. It's about supplementing our enjoyment of food with knowledge and mindfulness regarding its origins and effects.

It's about being flexible and compassionate with ourselves as we explore this plant-based lifestyle and recognizing that every plant-based meal is a step toward our green future.

Indeed, the ripples of our choices extend far beyond the personal. A green future redefines economies, fostering sustainable agricultural practices and encouraging local sourcing. It holds the potential to transform healthcare, as the decrease in preventable diseases alleviates the pressure on our systems.

And let's not overlook the social ripple effect, where our choices influence those around us, fostering communities that prioritize health and empathy.

And there it lies before us - a green future vibrant with possibility, where each of us holds the key to a treasure of wellness and worldly well-being.

Isn't it empowering to know that we can shape our destinies and contribute to a larger picture, a canvas that includes every living being and the very earth we walk upon?

As we close this chapter and look forward to turning fresh pages each day, let us hold onto this vision with both hands and hearts.

Together, let's welcome the dawn of a green future, a testament to the nourishing relationship we can foster with our bodies, communities, and the world. Sustainability, health, and compassion are ideals and choices we can (and should) make every time we eat. Here's to a future where our planet's bounty reflects our veins' vitality. Let's make it a reality, one plant-based bite at a time.

Appendix A: Recipe Inspirations for a Plant-Based Life

As we close this exploration of the astonishing benefits of a plant-based lifestyle, it's time to turn the theory into a delicious reality. You've learned about the vast spectrum of advantages, from the personal to the planetary, and now, the real fun begins.

You're ready to put on that apron and infuse your life with colors, flavors, and textures that satisfy the palate and fortify your health.

Embracing a plant-based diet isn't about munching on celery sticks or getting by on salads alone - far from it. It's a journey filled with many foods that most people never realize exist.

You're about to discover mouthwatering dishes that'll make you wonder why you didn't start eating this way sooner.

In this Appendix, I will give you a handful of yummy breakfast, lunch, snack, and dinner ideas to get you started. However, if you enjoyed this *Plant Diet Book*, please consider my vegan recipe book titled, "*51 Easy Plant-Based Meals: Delicious & Fantastic Vegan Recipes Anyone Can Make Quick.*" on www.Amazon.com

In that culinary treasure trove (*51 Easy Plant-Based Meals*), you'll find dozens of delectable recipes that are not only incredibly delicious but also easy to make. And while

you're on Amazon checking out that book, please take a
moment to let others know what you think about this book
on Amazon.

Your positive review will help others find this book. Plus, I
would truly love to hear how it has benefited you on your
plant-based journey.

If you point your smart phone camera at the QR code
below, it will give you a link to share your thoughts on
Amazon. Your positive feedback (and even a photo or
video of your copy with notes in it) can help other readers
also find this book.

Thank you so much for investing your valuable time here in
the pages of my book and giving your feedback, I truly
appreciate you.

Hearty Breakfasts to Kickstart Your Day

- Oatmeal and Porridges: Start with rolled oats or any whole grain, add a plant milk of your choice, some nuts, seeds, and your favorite fruits. Spice it up with cinnamon or nutmeg for a warming touch.

- Smoothie Bowl: Combine berries, bananas, and greens like spinach or kale in a blender, then pour into a bowl. Top it off with a handful of granola, seeds, and a drizzle of peanut butter.

- Everyday Smoothie: Don't toss out ugly, over-ripe bananas; instead, Freeze them in chunks before they go bad. Peel it, break it into thirds, and freeze it in a zip-lock bag. The following morning, combine several pieces of frozen banana in a blender with 2-3 dates (the number depends on how sweet you want it), add a large handful of fresh spinach, and fill with Almond Milk - this is your starting point or base. From here, you can add dairy-free chocolate chips for a chocolate smoothie or frozen berries (of your choice) for a delicious frozen drink each morning.

Wholesome Lunches That Pack a Punch

- Buddha Bowl: Layer brown rice or quinoa, an assortment of steamed or raw veggies, legumes like chickpeas or lentils, and a delicious tahini dressing.

- Wraps and Sandwiches: Stuff whole grain wraps with hummus, avocado, sliced veggies, beans, and greens. It's a portable meal that's perfect for on-the-go!

Dinners That Delight

- Stir-Fries: Sauté a medley of vegetables like bell peppers, broccoli, and carrots with tofu or tempeh in a splash of soy sauce and serve it over a bed of brown rice or noodles.

- Lentil Stews and Chilis: These are a great way to dip your toes into the world of legumes. They're hearty, satisfying, and chock-full of nutrients, perfect for a cozy night in.

Snacks for Sustained Energy

- Energy Balls: Mix oats, nut butter, a sweetener like maple syrup, and add-ins like chocolate chips or dried fruit. Roll into balls for a quick and nutritious snack.

- Crunchy Chickpeas: Roast chickpeas with your favorite spices until crispy for a satisfying, protein-rich snack.

Remember, these recipes are just a starting point. Feel free to experiment with ingredients and seasonings - a plant-based diet is incredibly versatile. You'll find you can create dishes that align with your health goals and your taste preferences.

Think of your kitchen as a laboratory where you can create meals that nourish and energize. It's about finding joy in your food while knowing you're doing something wonderful for your body and the world around you.

This appendix isn't meant to be a prescription but a source of inspiration.

Don't stress if a dish turns out wrong on the first try. Have fun with it, tweak as you go, and remember, the journey to a plant-strong life is as much about the adventure as the destination.

Welcome to a vibrant, plant-based life where every meal is an opportunity to do something good for yourself and the planet.

Appendix B: Nutritional Comparison Charts

By now, you've been armed with many insights into the mighty benefits of a plant-based diet. How do the actual numbers stack up? Let's take an illustrative dive into some nutritional comparison charts that offer clear, visual affirmations of why embracing plant power is a powerhouse move for your health.

Nutritional wisdom is about knowing what to eat and understanding how different foods impact the complex, beautiful machines we call bodies. If you find yourself debating the protein content in broccoli versus beef, you may wonder if spinach can truly stack up against salmon when it comes to iron. Well, let's lay those queries to rest.

Protein Punch: Plant vs. Animal

- **Soybean vs. Beef** - Soybeans offer slightly less protein per serving than beef but are rich in fiber, vitamins, minerals, and phytonutrients. Unlike beef, soybeans are cholesterol-free and lower in saturated fat, making them a healthier protein option, particularly for those concerned about cholesterol levels, and ideal for vegetarian or vegan diets.

- **Lentils vs. Chicken** - While chicken typically provides more protein per serving compared to lentils, it also contains saturated fat and cholesterol, whereas lentils are high in fiber, vitamins, minerals, and phytonutrients, making them a nutritious plant-based protein option with additional health benefits.

- **Quinoa vs. Pork** - Quinoa offers a more nutrient-dense and heart-healthy option due to its higher fiber content, lower saturated fat content, and absence of cholesterol.

- **Tofu vs. Eggs** - Per serving, tofu typically provides about the same amount of protein compared to eggs but without the cholesterol, or potential health hazards of eating animal proteins.

Here's a little spoiler: when you compare calorie for calorie, many plant-based protein sources bring more to the table than just amino acids. They're hosting a party, and fiber, vitamins, and minerals are all on the guest list - without the saturated fat and cholesterol that often crash animal protein gatherings.

Omega Waves: Fatty Acid Faceoff

Flaxseeds vs. Salmon

- Flaxseeds are one of the richest plant sources of Alpha-Linolenic Acid (ALA), an essential Omega-3 fatty acid. ALA is converted in the body to eicosapentaenoic acid (EPA) and docosahexaenoic acid (DHA), although this conversion process is limited in efficiency. ALA is known for its anti-inflammatory properties and potential cardiovascular benefits.

- Flaxseeds also contain Omega-6 fatty acids, such as linoleic acid (LA), in smaller amounts compared to ALA. Omega-6 fatty acids play a role in maintaining healthy cell membranes and supporting immune function.

- Flaxseeds contain small amounts of Omega-9 fatty acids (such as oleic acid), which are monounsaturated fats known for their potential cardiovascular benefits.

Flaxseeds are rich in ALA, while salmon provides EPA and DHA directly (and unwanted cholesterol and mercury).

Chia Seeds vs. Tuna

- Chia seeds are one of the richest plant sources of ALA (an essential omega-3 fatty acid). ALA is converted in the body to eicosapentaenoic acid (EPA) and docosahexaenoic acid (DHA), although this conversion process is limited in efficiency. ALA is known for its anti-inflammatory properties and potential cardiovascular benefits.

- Chia seeds contain Omega-6 fatty acids, such as linoleic acid (LA), in smaller amounts compared to ALA. Omega-6 fatty acids play a role in maintaining healthy cell membranes and supporting immune function.

- Chia seeds contain some Omega-9 fatty acids, such as oleic acid, which are monounsaturated fats known for their potential cardiovascular benefits.

Chia seeds are rich in ALA, while tuna provides EPA and DHA directly without cholesterol and mercury.

Walnuts vs. Cod Liver Oil

- Walnuts are one of the richest plant sources of ALA, an essential Omega-3 fatty acid. ALA is converted in the body to eicosapentaenoic acid (EPA) and docosahexaenoic acid (DHA), although this conversion process is limited in efficiency. ALA is known for its anti-inflammatory properties and potential cardiovascular benefits.

- Walnuts contain Omega-6 fatty acids, such as linoleic acid (LA), in smaller amounts compared to ALA. Omega-6 fatty acids play a role in maintaining healthy cell membranes and supporting immune function.

- Walnuts contain some Omega-9 fatty acids, such as oleic acid, which are monounsaturated fats known for their potential cardiovascular benefits.

Walnuts are rich in ALA, while cod liver oil provides EPA and DHA directly without cholesterol and only trace amounts of mercury

Hemp Seeds vs. Mackerel

- Hemp seeds are rich in ALA, an essential Omega-3 fatty acid. ALA is converted in the body to eicosapentaenoic acid (EPA) and docosahexaenoic acid (DHA), although this conversion process is limited in efficiency. ALA is known for its anti-inflammatory properties and potential cardiovascular benefits.

- Hemp seeds contain linoleic acid, an Omega-6 fatty acid that is essential for maintaining healthy cell membranes and supporting immune function.

- Hemp seeds contain some Omega-9 fatty acids, such as oleic acid, which are monounsaturated fats known for their potential cardiovascular benefits.

Hemp seeds are rich in ALA, while mackerel provides EPA and DHA directly without cholesterol and mercury.

Dive into the Omega-3 scene where plant-based contenders like flaxseeds and chia seeds show us they're no underdogs. Without the mercury worries of fish, these seeds deliver Omega-3s gracefully and leave the oceanic ecosystem undisturbed.

Iron Isles: A Mineral Melee

- **Spinach vs. Red Meat** - While both spinach and red meat contain iron, red meat provides heme iron, which is more easily absorbed by the body compared to the non-heme iron found in spinach. However, spinach offers additional nutrients and is a valuable source of iron for individuals following vegetarian or vegan diets. Consuming a variety of iron-rich foods, along with vitamin C-rich foods to enhance non-heme iron absorption, can help meet daily iron requirements and support overall health.

- **Lentils vs. Pork** - while both lentils and pork contain iron, pork provides heme iron, which is more easily absorbed by the body compared to the non-heme iron found in lentils. However, lentils offer additional nutrients and are a valuable source of iron for individuals following vegetarian or vegan diets. Consuming a variety of iron-rich foods, along with vitamin C-rich foods to enhance non-heme iron absorption, can help meet daily iron requirements and support overall health.

- **Soybeans vs. Chicken Liver** - While both soybeans and chicken liver contain iron, chicken liver provides heme iron, which is more easily absorbed by the body compared to the non-heme iron found in soybeans. However, soybeans offer additional nutrients and are a valuable source of iron for individuals following vegetarian or vegan diets. Consuming a variety of iron-rich foods, along with vitamin C-rich foods to enhance non-heme iron absorption, can help meet daily iron requirements and support overall health.

- **Chickpeas vs. Lamb** - While both chickpeas and lamb contain iron, lamb provides heme iron, which is more easily absorbed by the body compared to the non-heme iron found in chickpeas. However, chickpeas offer additional nutrients and are a valuable source of iron for individuals following vegetarian or vegan diets. Consuming a variety of iron-rich foods, along with vitamin C-rich foods to enhance non-heme iron absorption, can help meet daily iron requirements and support overall health.

While iron from plants (non-heme iron) often bears the rap of being less absorbable, it comes without the baggage linked to the heme iron found in meats: no associations with certain types of heart problems or diabetes. That being said, if you consume it with vitamin C-rich foods, this can help with absorption.

The chart may show that animal sources appear higher in iron, but when you account for the incredible cruelty involved with killing these animals for food or the nutrient-rich content of plants that star in other health-promoting roles, it's clear who the true heroes are.

Calcium Castles: Building Strong Bones

Almond Milk vs. Cow's Milk

- Almond milk is typically lower in calories compared to cow's milk, making it a suitable option for those watching their calorie intake.

- Almond milk is naturally dairy-free, making it an excellent alternative for individuals who are lactose intolerant or have dairy allergies.

- Many commercially available almond milks are fortified with vitamins and minerals, including calcium, vitamin D, and vitamin E, making them comparable to cow's milk in terms of nutritional content.

- Almond milk is naturally cholesterol-free and low in saturated fat, which contributes to heart health when consumed as part of a balanced diet.

- Almond milk is a good source of vitamin E, an antioxidant that supports immune function and skin health. It also contains healthy fats, such as monounsaturated fats, which may help reduce the risk of heart disease.

Kale vs. Cheese

- Kale is a leafy green vegetable that contains a significant amount of calcium per serving. While kale's calcium content varies depending on factors like variety and preparation method, it is considered an excellent plant-based source of calcium.

- The calcium in kale is accompanied by oxalates, compounds that can bind to calcium and reduce its absorption in the body. However, kale is also rich in vitamin C, which can enhance calcium absorption. Cooking kale can also help reduce its oxalate content, potentially improving calcium bioavailability.

- In addition to calcium, kale is rich in other essential nutrients, including vitamin K, vitamin C, vitamin A, fiber, and antioxidants. These nutrients contribute to bone health, immune function, and overall well-being.

- Kale is low in calories and carbohydrates, making it a nutrient-dense food that can be incorporated into a variety of dishes to boost calcium intake without significantly increasing calorie consumption.

Tofu vs. Yogurt

- Tofu is made from soybeans, and depending on the coagulant used and the processing method, it can contain varying amounts of calcium. Tofu is often fortified with calcium to enhance its nutritional value, especially for those who follow a plant-based diet.

- The calcium in tofu is bound to oxalates, compounds that can inhibit calcium absorption. However, tofu is also rich in other nutrients, such as magnesium and phosphorus, which can help counteract the effects of oxalates and improve calcium absorption.

- Tofu provides a calcium-rich alternative to dairy products for individuals who are lactose intolerant, allergic to dairy, or following a vegan or vegetarian diet.

Tofu is a plant-based source of calcium that may contain fortified calcium, while yogurt provides calcium along with probiotics and other nutrients and problems related to dairy consumption. Including a variety of calcium-rich foods in the diet, such as tofu, yogurt, leafy greens, and fortified foods, can help meet daily calcium needs and support bone health.

Did you know that plant-based sources of calcium like kale and almonds come packaged with antioxidants and do not bring along the saturated fat often found in their dairy counterparts?

They're crafting bone health on a foundation of holistic goodness.

You should also know that cow's milk is designed for baby cows, not humans. Humans should not consume dairy (cow's milk, dairy cheese, or butter) for the same reason you would not want a transfusion of cow's blood: You're not a bovine.

Many plant-based milk alternatives, such as almond, soy, and oat milk, offer similar nutrients without the potential drawbacks associated with cow's milk.

Individuals concerned about the health implications of cow's milk should consult with a healthcare professional or registered dietitian for personalized dietary guidance.

And speaking of the concerns or health implications of consuming dairy (cow's milk, butter, and cheese), take a look at this list of related problems:

Problems With Consuming Dairy

Lactose Intolerance: Many individuals worldwide have lactose intolerance, a condition where the body lacks the enzyme lactase needed to digest lactose, the sugar found in dairy milk. Symptoms of lactose intolerance include bloating, gas, diarrhea, and abdominal discomfort after consuming milk or dairy products.

Allergies: Cow's milk allergy is one of the most common food allergies, particularly in infants and young children. Symptoms can range from mild, such as hives and digestive issues, to severe, including difficulty breathing and anaphylaxis.

Saturated Fat and Cholesterol: Whole milk and dairy products can be high in saturated fat and cholesterol, which are linked to an increased risk of heart disease, stroke, and other cardiovascular issues when consumed in excess.

Bone Health and Osteoporosis: Contrary to popular belief, some research suggests that high consumption of animal protein, including milk protein, may actually increase calcium excretion from the bones, potentially weakening them over time.

Additionally, countries with the highest dairy consumption often have the highest rates of osteoporosis.

Cancer: Some studies have suggested a potential link between dairy consumption and certain cancers, such as prostate and ovarian cancer.

Hormones and Antibiotics: Commercial dairy farming often involves the use of growth hormones and antibiotics to increase milk production and prevent diseases. Concerns have been raised about the health effects of these substances when consumed by humans.

Ethical and Environmental Concerns: Dairy farming practices, including confinement housing and the separation of calves from their mothers shortly after birth, have raised ethical concerns. Additionally, the environmental impact of dairy production, including greenhouse gas emissions and water usage, has raised sustainability concerns as well.

Summary

A visual tour of these charts makes it crystal clear that opting for plants over animal products isn't just about matching nutrient for nutrient; it's choosing foods rich in life-promoting properties that go beyond mere numbers.

Yes, plants have protein, iron, omega-3s, and calcium covered. But they also bring peace of mind, knowing that what's on your plate fosters health for your body and the planet.

So, take a gander at these charts. Let them reassure you as they illustrate the incredible potential resting at the tip of your fork, ready to nourish, sustain, and rejuvenate you. That's the beauty of a plant-based diet - it's a choice packed with potent nutrients, backed by science, and kind to all.

Appendix C: Resources for Further Reading

Taking the final turn towards a plant-based lifestyle isn't just about what you stock in your fridge or pile onto your plate; it's about enriching your mind with knowledge to bolster your confidence in this life-changing decision.

As you've journeyed through these chapters and explored the diet of early humans throughout history, you might wonder, "Now what, what's next?"

As you have discovered in this book, adopting a plant-based diet is a lifestyle change encompassing many things like our biology, nutrition, and the social aspects of eating.

Knowing where to turn next or how to get started doesn't have to be complicated or confusing. More insights, data, and what to eat to strengthen your resolve and understanding can be easily discovered.

Let's cultivate that budding interest with a curated list of resources. Here, you'll find books, articles, and papers that will expand your horizons and provide ammunition for those dinner table debates or the quiet pondering in the comfort of your nook.

Books to Flip Through

- *Whole: Rethinking the Science of Nutrition* - is one of the most profound books on this subject that I have ever read; it offers a comprehensive and compelling exploration of the link between nutrition and health, challenging readers to reconsider their dietary habits and adopt a more plant-based approach to eating for long-term well-being.

- *World Peace Diet: Eating for Spiritual Health and Social Harmony* - The World Peace Diet suggests how we as a species might move our consciousness forward so that we can be more free, more intelligent, more loving, and happier in the choices we make.

- *The Omnivore's Dilemma* – Dive into this investigation of food chains and the impact of our eating habits on our health and the planet.

- *Eating Animals* – Explore the ethical and personal questions surrounding our food choices and the journey from farm to plate.

- *The China Study* – Learn about one of the most comprehensive studies on nutrition ever conducted and its implications on long-term health.

- *How Not to Die* – Discover foods scientifically proven to prevent and reverse disease, emphasizing a plant-based diet's benefits.

- *Food and Mood* – Understand the profound ways that food choices can affect our brains, behavior, and emotions.

Scientific Journals & Articles

For those who crave the hard-hitting facts, there's a garden of scholarly articles waiting to be harvested. Scientific journals like *The American Journal of Clinical Nutrition*, *Nutrition Reviews*, and *The Lancet*, to name a few, are packed with peer-reviewed articles that delve deep into the effects of plant-based diets on various aspects of health and disease prevention. Websites like PubMed and ScienceDirect can be your starting point to unearth these writings.

Documentaries to Watch

If a picture is worth a thousand words, then documentaries might just be priceless, particularly those that provide visual evidence to support the health claims of a plant-based diet. Here are a few to consider:

1. **Cowspiracy: The Sustainability Secret -** *Follow the shocking, yet humorous, journey of an aspiring environmentalist, as he daringly seeks to find the real solution to the most pressing environmental issues and true path to sustainability.*

2. **Forks Over Knives** – Examines the profound claim that most, if not all, of the degenerative diseases that afflict us can be controlled, or even reversed, by rejecting our present menu of animal-based and processed foods.

3. **Dominion** - uses drones, hidden and handheld cameras to expose the dark

underbelly of modern animal agriculture, questioning the morality and validity of humankind's dominion over the animal kingdom.

4. **Eating Our Way to Extinction** - Alarming and entertaining this compelling feature documentary will make you never look at your food or the food industry in the same way again.

5. **What the Health** – An intrepid filmmaker on a journey of discovery as he uncovers possibly the largest health secret of our time and the collusion between industry, government, pharmaceutical and health organizations keeping this information from us.

6. **The Game Changers** – A UFC fighter's world is turned upside down when he discovers an elite group of world-renowned athletes and scientists who prove that everything he had been taught about protein was a lie.

7. **Eating Animals** - An examination of our dietary choices and the food we put in our bodies.

8. **Vegucated** - is a guerrilla-style documentary that follows three meat- and cheese-loving New Yorkers who agree to adopt a vegan diet for six weeks and learn what it's all about.

9. **Earthlings** - Using hidden cameras and never-before-seen footage, Earthlings chronicles the day-to-day practices of the largest industries in the world, all of which rely entirely on animals for profit.

10. **Fat, Sick & Nearly Dead** - is an American documentary that chronicles Australian Joe Cross's 60-day journey across the United States, where he embarks on a juice-only fast in a quest to reclaim his health.

Remember, the journey of healthier eating and living isn't a solo adventure. It's a road shared by many, backed by research, and trodden by those seeking vigor and vitality.

As you explore these resources, your path becomes clearer and your commitment to a plant-based future stronger. Keep reading, keep learning, and let your curiosity about plant-based eating blossom into informed confidence.

This has been,
"Plant Diet Book: Why Your Body Prefers Plants".
Written by Robert Enochs
Copyright 2026 by Robert Enochs

For some delicious recipes to try, please consider one of his cook books, *"51 Easy Plant-Based Meals: Delicious & Fantastic Vegan Recipes Anyone Can Make Quick"*

If you'd like to contact Robert or check out other books he's written, please visit www.RobertEnochs.com